Jack Hadley, a senior research associate with The Urban Institute's Center for Health Policy, received his doctorate in economics from Yale University. He is the coauthor of *Insuring the Nation's Health* and editor of *Medical Education Financing*.

More Medical Care, Better Health?

An Economic Analysis of Mortality Rates

Jack Hadley

An Urban Institute Book

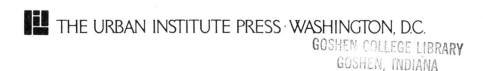 THE URBAN INSTITUTE PRESS · WASHINGTON, D.C.

Research support for this book was
provided by Grant No. 5-R01-HS-
02790 from the National Center for
Health Services Research, Office of the
Assistant Secretary for Health, Department of Health and Human Services,
and by the Ford Foundation.

THE URBAN INSTITUTE is a nonprofit policy research and educational organization established in Washington, D.C. in 1968. Its staff investigates interrelated social and economic problems of urban communities and government policies affecting those communities and the people who live in them. The Institute disseminates significant findings of such research through the active publications program of its Press. The Institute has two goals for work in each of its research areas: to help shape thinking about societal problems and efforts to solve them, and to improve government decisions and performance by providing better information and analytic tools.

Through work that ranges from broad conceptual studies to administrative and technical assistance, Institute researchers contribute to the stock of knowledge available to public officials and to private individuals and groups concerned with formulating and implementing more efficient and effective government policy.

Conclusions or opinions expressed are those of the authors and do not necessarily reflect the views of other staff members, officers, or trustees of the Institute, or of any organizations which provide financial support to the Institute.

CONTENTS

TABLES

FIGURES

MAPS

FOREWORD

Most of the recent debate over public spending for health care has focused on its cost—the share of GNP devoted to health care; the rate of increase in health care spending per capita; or the price of a day in the hospital. The important question of medical care's actual impact on health is rarely addressed, partly because good evidence of the effect of medical care has not been available.

This book, however, closes the gap left in previous analyses of public health needs and policies. *More Medical Care, Better Health?* reports the results of a detailed statistical analysis of the relationship between mortality rates and medical care use and demonstrates that, contrary to the conventional wisdom of the analytic community, more medical care use does appear to lower mortality rates. Furthermore, the author shows that knowledge of the relationship between medical care use and mortality rates clarifies the complicated issues of deciding how much to spend on medical care, what to buy, and how to evaluate various pro-health policies.

This analysis of mortality rates is part of The Urban Institute Health Policy Center's program to explore issues in health policy and health financing. The Center's research staff of fifteen economists, political scientists, and other policy analysts has conducted numerous studies of the effects of alternative payment mechanisms on service delivery by hospitals, physicians, nursing homes, and home-care providers; of the design of policies to finance acute and long-term care at acceptable public and private expense; and of the health care politics and law that establish the environment in which public policies are made. Through studies like Hadley's, the Health Policy Center aims to contribute to the continuing debate on balancing the value of medical care with its cost, and on structuring appropriate roles for the private sector and state, local, and federal governments in financing service, promoting efficiency, and maintaining adequate access to care.

The author thanks the many people who contributed to the study. John Holahan, Judith Feder, Robert Lee, Michael Grossman, Kenneth Warner, Joel Kleinman, David Rabin, Roger Cole, and L. Jack Rodgers read

drafts and made useful comments. Cathy Carlson, Anthony Osei, and
Patricia Tigue provided skilled research assistance. Jacob Feldman of the
National Center for Health Statistics granted access to the detailed mortality data. Elizabeth Beach and Gwen Stanley of Group Operations Inc.
constructed the computer files used in the analysis. Alfred Meltzer and
Colleen Goodman of Applied Management Sciences put together an expanded version of the Area Resource File to meet the needs of this study.
Martina Pass and Johnetta Ward diligently and cheerfully typed the bulk
of the manuscript. Finally, Lih Y. Young of The National Center for
Health Services Research was a thoughtful and patient project officer who
provided both intellectual and administrative support.

William Gorham
President
The Urban Institute

More
Medical Care,
Better Health?

1

HEALTH AND PUBLIC POLICY

The attainment and maintenance of good health have long been accepted societal objectives. Good health is valued in its own right as an important component of individual well-being. In addition, health is significant in the level of economic activity it generates through its effects on labor force participation, the supply of healthy work days, worker productivity, and direct expenditures for medical services.[1] The U.S. Department of Health and Human Services (DHHS) has defined the nation's health objectives by announcing 20 explicit goals for disease prevention, health promotion, and health status outcomes.[2] For example, the infant mortality rate should be less than 12 per 1,000 live births; the death rate for adults between 25 and 64 years old should be less than 5 per 1,000 people; and for those 65 and older, the age-adjusted average number of days of restricted activity per year due to acute and chronic conditions should be less than 30 per person.[3]

Given that attaining and maintaining good health are legitimate public policy goals, the question of what are the best strategies for reaching these targets becomes important. The range of potential policy options is extensive. It includes changing the quantity and mix of medical care services, promoting health-enhancing behavior, increasing income transfers, conducting educational activities, reducing pollution, improving job safety, and placing greater controls on toxic and radioactive substances. In order to choose among these policies, officials need better information on each policy's cost and potential impact on health.

The conceptual cornerstone of the research reported in this book is an analogy between the processes which determine health levels and the economic theory of production. According to this analogy, health is the output which is produced by combining medical care, personal behavior,

1

socioeconomic conditions, environmental factors, and hereditary/biological factors. These health-determining elements are akin to inputs in the production process. As such, each makes some contribution, positive or negative, to the level of output (health), and each has some cost associated with a change in its level.

Policies aimed at improving health should take into account the nature of the health production function and the costs of its inputs. The specific objectives of this study follow from this general goal. The first is to investigate the relationship between the use of medical care and various infant and adult mortality rates. (Mortality rates are used as health indicators throughout the study.) The second objective is to examine the contributions of income and education to variations in mortality rates. The third objective is to demonstrate and illustrate how information from the health production function can be applied to the problems of designating medically underserved areas and reallocating medical care services.

Interest in these issues is motivated by reasons besides the importance of good health to economic and social well-being. For one, there is a growing body of opinion that additional medical care use is no longer significant in the health of the nation. According to Victor Fuchs, ". . . when the state of medical science and other health-determining variables are held constant, the marginal contribution of medical care to health is very small in modern nations."[4] This belief was prompted in part by the distinct leveling off of age-adjusted mortality rates, particularly for males, between 1950 and 1970. As shown in table 1, for example, the mortality rate for white males declined by 17 percent between 1940 and 1950, but by only 3.6 percent per decade between 1950 and 1970. Nonwhite males actually experienced an increased mortality rate between 1960 and 1970. To a large extent, the period of near-static mortality rates coincided with significant increases in medical care consumption, which increased from 4.5 to 7.2 percent of GNP between 1950 and 1970.[5] After adjusting for inflation, per capita consumption of medical care increased by almost 75 percent, from $109 per person in 1950 to $187 in 1970. The belief that additional medical care is no longer an important contributor to improved health is further buttressed by concerns over iatrogenic disease and the medical capability to prolong life for nonfunctioning, terminally ill persons.[6] Finally, the results of several statistical studies imply that additional medical care use may have no significant impact on either mortality or morbidity.[7]

More recent experience, however, suggests that these conclusions may be premature. Since 1970, mortality rates have been dropping at an increasing rate. The age-adjusted mortality rate for the entire population

TABLE 1

Percentage Changes in Death Rates By Age, Race, and Sex,
United States, 1940-1978

	All Ages[a]	Age				
		45-54	55-64	65-74	75-84	85+
White Male						
1940-1950	−0.17	−0.14	−0.09	−0.11	−0.14	−0.12
1950-1960	−0.04	−0.50	−0.03	−0.00*	−0.02	−0.02
1960-1970	−0.03	−0.50	−0.01	−0.01	−0.02	−0.15
1970-1978	−0.14	−0.16	−0.18	−0.14	−0.02	−0.03
White Female						
1940-1950	−0.26	−0.27	−0.23	−0.22	−0.19	−0.16
1950-1960	−0.14	−0.16	−0.16	−0.14	−0.09	−0.01
1960-1970	−0.11	0.00	−0.06	−0.11	−0.13	−0.18
1970-1978	−0.14	−0.13	−0.08	−0.17	−0.14	−0.04
All Other, Male						
1940-1950	−0.23	−0.24	−0.06	−0.08	−0.17	−0.20
1950-1960	−0.11	−0.17	−0.09	−0.02	−0.04	−0.05
1960-1970	0.02	0.06	−0.03	−0.03	−0.04	−0.25
1970-1978	−0.16	−0.24	−0.12	−0.18	−0.00*	−0.11
All Other, Female						
1940-1950	−0.27	−0.27	−0.17	−0.12	−0.16	−0.16
1950-1960	−0.18	−0.26	−0.13	−0.14	−0.05	−0.04
1960-1970	−0.13	−0.14	−0.22	−0.08	−0.05	−0.20
1970-1978	−0.21	−0.32	−0.17	−0.26	−0.00*	−0.16
Total Population						
1940-1950	−0.22	−0.20	−0.14	−0.15	−0.17	−0.14
1950-1960	−0.10	−0.11	−0.08	−0.07	−0.06	−0.02
1960-1970	−0.07	−0.04	−0.05	−0.06	−0.09	−0.18
1970-1978	−0.14	−0.16	−0.15	−0.16	−0.11	−0.10

*Less than −.005 percent.
a. Age-adjusted.

declined 14 percent between 1970 and 1978, twice the decline between
1960 and 1970. This trend also coincided with significant increases in
medical care use, particularly by beneficiaries of the federal medical care
initiatives of the late 1960s (Medicare, Medicaid, Maternal and Child
Health, Neighborhood Health Centers, etc.). In addition, there are several
statistical analyses which suggest that medical care does have the expected
negative effect on illness.[8]

Thus, the issue of the impact of additional medical care use on health is
far from conclusively resolved. What does seem clear is that simple com-

parisons of trends in mortality rates and medical care expenditures may be very misleading guides for public policy toward medical care spending and use.

The second factor motivating this research is recent findings regarding the effects of income and education on mortality. As with the medical care-mortality relationship, there is growing opinion and evidence that increasing income does not result in better health. Again quoting Victor Fuchs, "... in the United States the relation between income and life expectancy has tended to disappear."[9] This contradicts one of the most common findings of early (pre-1960) research on the determinants of variations in mortality rates. Explanations of the income-mortality paradox include a positive income elasticity of demand for unhealthy goods and activities, the existence of a natural limit on the ability of living standards to improve health, deleterious health consequence as byproducts of activities which generate high incomes, and the statistical inability to untangle the effects of income from education. Since much of this research has been based upon highly aggregated data, this issue also needs further investigation.

The final factor motivating this study is the growing controversy over planning and direct government intervention as mechanisms for allocating medical care resources. A good example of this approach is the designation of health manpower shortage areas by the U.S. Department of Health and Human Services. Designated areas are eligible to apply for physicians from the National Health Service Corps (NHSC), a federal program which employs physicians and other health professionals. To date, the main criterion for designating shortage areas has been the ratio of physicians to population in a county. Areas with fewer than one nonfederal, full-time equivalent primary care physician per 3,500 people are generally eligible to become NHSC sites.[10]

This criterion has a number of obvious flaws: the contributions of other medical care resources are ignored; there is no direct link between the criterion and any measure of health; the border-crossing problem is not dealt with adequately; and the designation ratio is both arbitrary and inflexible.[11] An alternative approach to evaluating the distribution of physicians (or other medical care resources) is to use the information implicit in the health production function. In particular, knowledge of physicians' marginal productivity in reducing mortality suggests several criteria for determining the optimal distribution of physicians.[12] Thus, the project's final objective is to develop alternative estimates of manpower shortages and optimal physician distribution in order to compare them to estimates based on existing methods.

Study Design

The primary task of this study is estimation of a series of health production functions using aggregate, cross-sectional data for 1970. (1970 is the study year in order to take advantage of data from the 1970 Census of Population and from special mortality files created under the sponsorship of the National Center for Health Statistics (NCHS).) Although several of the issues just discussed are couched in terms of changes over time, analysis of cross-sectional data nevertheless provides useful information and in some respects may be superior to analysis of time-series data. For example, cross-sectional variations in mortality rates, medical care resource availability, income, and education generally parallel or exceed time-series variations. This should facilitate the statistical analysis. A second advantage of a single cross-section is that it holds constant much of the impact of changes in medical knowledge and technology. The post-World War II period has been marked by dramatic changes in medical techniques, equipment, and knowlege. These changes cannot be measured very well. Using information from a single period provides a better opportunity to identify the effects of variations in medical care use on mortality rates.

This study extends earlier research on health production functions by using a more disaggregated and refined data set than analyzed in other studies. First, the unit of analysis is the county group, as defined by the Census Bureau. County groups consist of one or more whole counties with a minimum population of 250,000 people, The criteria for grouping counties are similar to those used to designate state economic areas. However, a county group can encompass counties in more than one state.

There were over 400 county groups in 1970, thus providing many more observations than are available with state analysis. Further, the extent of intraunit heterogeneity with regard to area conditions and population characteristics is likely to be less than for states. Compared to the individual county, the county group has two advantages: it has a reasonably large minimum population; and it is constructed to conform to local economic and market patterns. The latter lessens the problems associated with the artificiality of a political boundary (e.g., a county line) as a constraint on population activites. Finally, unlike most standard metropolitan statistical areas (SMSAs), a number of county groups are composed largely of small urban and rural communities. Thus the experiences of these areas are not excluded from the analysis.

A second extension from earlier research is this study's focus on age-sex-race-specific mortality rates for eight adult and four infant population cohorts. The particular cohorts analyzed are as follows:

White males, 45 to 64 years old
Black males, 45 to 64 years old
White females, 45 to 64 years old
Black females, 45 to 64 years old
White males, 65 and older
Black males, 65 and older
White females, 65 and older
Black females, 65 and older
White male infants (less than 1 year old)
Black male infants (less than 1 year old)
White female infants (less than 1 year old)
Black female infants (less than 1 year old)

Together, these cohorts account for more than 90 percent of all deaths. Cohort-specific analyses also provide a direct method of controlling for many of the effects of age, sex, and race on mortality without having to make any explicit assumptions about the nature of those effects.

Detailed data on the socioeconomic characteristics of each cohort are based on a 2 percent sample of individuals from the 1970 Census. The data for each county group are constructed by aggregating individual's characteristics within each population cohort. As a result, there is a very close correspondence between the population underlying the measurement of the mortality rates and the population underlying the construction of the sociodemographic variables. This is particularly true for the income, education, occupation, and family status variables which are generally not available from published sources in the required population break-downs. (Information on infant mortality rates is matched with characteristics of women of child-bearing age, 14 to 44, in each county group.)

Finally, all mortality data are drawn from the National Center for Health Statisics' vital statistics. Deaths by age, sex, and race for more than 40 individual causes and disease groups are taken from death certificates based on decedents' county of residence for all deaths which occurred over a 4.5 year period (1968 through the first half of 1972). Infant mortality data cover the five-year period, 1969 to 1973. Combining several years' death records has the advantage of lessening the effects of truly random events, such as local epidemics or natural disasters which occur in only one year. The mortality data are also aggregated to the county group level and linked with data from the 1970 Census and from a variety of other secondary sources to create the final analysis file.

The remainder of this book is divided into eight sections: theory, literature review, empirical methods, results for the adult cohorts, results for the infant cohorts, the effects of income and education, policy applications, and summary and conclusions. The theory chapter describes the relationships underlying the specification of the health production function. In its most general form the theory of health production posits that health is a function of enivironmental, behavioral, hereditary, and medical care factors. However, in this form the theory has little analytic content. Therefore, following Grossman, we hypothesize that the health production function is part of a larger model which includes relationships for the demand for health and the demand for and supply of medical care.[13] The advantage of this approach is that it provides a clear rationale for the existence of a health production function and an explicit statement of endogenous and exogenous variables.

The literature review provides a brief summary of earlier analyses of geographic variations in both adult and infant mortality rates. Its objectives are twofold: to identify variables which ought to be included in the health production function specifications, and to highlight areas where further research is needed. The empirical methods chapter describes the steps required to move from the theory to the empirical model. Issues covered are the use of the mortality rate as a proxy for health and the choice of a measure of medical care use or resources. (Appendix A discusses the choice of functional form, provides detailed information on data sources and variable definitions, and explores several econometric issues.)

The report's next three chapters present the major empirical results of the study. Chapter 5 focuses on adult mortality rates from all causes and from several major disease-specific causes of death. Chapter 6 considers infant mortality rates, with separate results reported for the neonatal and postneonatal phases of infancy. In chapter 7 we examine the relationships among income, education, and mortality rates. Two questions are considered: do various components of total family income have differential effects on mortality rates, and can the independent effects of income and education be identified?

In chapter 8, we turn to the implications of the health production function estimates for the geographic distribution of medical care. Two potential policy questions are raised. What would be the impact on mortality rates of an across-the-board 10 percent increase in medical care use? How many more physicians would be needed in order to lower above-average, cohort-specific mortality rates to the national average for each cohort in 1970? The results of these policy simulations are then used to construct criteria for ranking counties in terms of medical care shortage. These rankings are then compared to a ranking based on the ratio of population to physicians. The report's final chapter summarizes the study's methods and major findings. Recommendations are made for both policy and future research.

Summary of Major Findings

The principal finding of this study is that medical care use has a negative and statistically significant impact on mortality rates. This implies that health is better when medical care use is higher. After controlling for other factors, such as income, education, marital status, work experience, cigarette consumption, and disability, cohorts with greater estimated use of medical care appear to have lower mortality rates (for all causes of death). Except for middle-aged males (45 to 64 years old), the magnitude of the relationship between the mortality rate and medical care use is surprisingly similar across cohorts. A 10 percent increase in medical care expenditures per capita is estimated to reduce mortality rates by between 1.23 percent (elderly white males) and 2.04 percent (black female infants), with an average reduction of 1.57 percent. The estimated impact is largest for white middle-aged males, 3.24 percent, and smallest for black middle-aged males, 0.77 percent. Again excepting middle-aged males, the effect of an increase in medical care use appears to be slightly larger, by about 25 percent, for blacks in each of the age-sex cohorts studied. Overall, these results suggest that even though average mortality rates and average medical care expenditures per capita vary greatly by age, sex, and race, the effect of a small increase in expenditures per capita on mortality rates is fairly similar across population groups.

Exploratory analysis of cause-specific mortality rates reinforces the basic finding of a negative relationship between medical care use and mortality. Adult deaths were grouped into four cause-specific categories: external causes, cancers, ischemic heart diseases, and cardiovascular diseases. Over the last 10 years, the largest decreases in adult mortality rates have occurred in the ischemic heart and cardiovascular disease categories; the death rate from external causes has declined slightly; and the cancer death rate has remained essentially static. Estimates of the impact of medical care drawn from cause-specific health production functions estimated with cross-sectional data for 1970 are highly consistent with these trends. The largest estimated effect of an increase in medical care use occurs in the ischemic heart and cardiovascular diseases mortality rates.

However, except for white middle-aged males, the use of medical care does not have a statistically significant and negative effect on mortality rates from either external causes or cancer.

Both higher incomes and higher educational attainment are also generally associated with lower mortality rates. However, the nature of the relationship between these factors and mortality rates is much more complex than the medical care-mortality relationship. In particular, the effect of income on mortality depends on the age group considered, the type of income, and the interrelationship with education. Higher educational attainment is more consistently associated than income with lower mortality rates. However, the magnitude of education's effect depends on whether income is included in the production function.

A family's total income has a larger and generally statistically significant association with infant mortality than with adult mortality. For adults, the association varies with both type of income and age. Pure transfer payments from both public and private sources generally have a negative and statistically significant relationship with mortality rates of all adult cohorts. Earned income, however, tends to have a negative association with mortality rates of working age (45 to 64 years old) cohorts, but a positive association with mortality rates of elderly cohorts. Unearned income, which includes the earnings of other family members as well as transfer payments, appears to have effects opposite those of earned income. These results suggest that the income-mortality relationship depends closely on the interactions between health status, the ability to work, and the need to work.

Finally, estimates of the magnitude and statistical significance of the effects of education and income on mortality rates do depend critically on whether one or both of the factors are included in the health production function. When only one of the two is included, its impact is generally larger in magnitude (by about 50 percent) and more likely to be statistically significant than when both variables are in the function. Overall, then, the results indicate that while it is difficult to identify the effects of income and education on mortality rates with precision, the relationships are generally inverse, that is, higher incomes and education levels are associated with lower mortality rates.

The final phase of the analysis investigates and illustrates how the health production function can be used to address health policy issues. Three general policy questions are explored. Which counties should be designated as having medical care shortages? How many additional physicians are needed in the U.S.? How does increasing medical care use compare to other policies to reduce mortality rates? In each policy analysis, the health production function estimates are used to compute how the mortality rate would change if medical care expenditures, or another policy variable, were changed with all other factors held fixed. Combining the change in the mortality rate with information on the cost of changing the value of the input (policy) variable results in an estimate of the cost of averting a death under alternative approaches and in different locations. These estimates of the cost of averting a death are the foundation of the policy analyses.

The process of designating counties which need additional medical care resources is based on the assumption that the policy maker wishes to maximize the number of deaths averted for a specified increase in medical care spending. Using the estimate of the cost-per-death-averted derived from the health production function, counties are ranked on the basis of the number of deaths which would be averted per $100,000 increase in medical care consumption by county residents. Allocating additional medical care resources to the counties with the largest number of deaths averted would satisfy the policy's goal.

The number of deaths averted per $100,000 increase in medical care consumption is, of course, only one possible criterion for ranking counties in terms of medical underservice or the need for additional medical care. Several current programs rely primarily on the population-per-primary-care-physician (POPPC) ratio to designate eligibility for government assistance. How closely related are these two criteria? Computing the simple correlation between the values of these two ranking criteria for all U.S. counties suggests only a small, positive association ($\rho = 0.18$). This lack of correspondence is reinforced by examining the 500 "most needy" counties under each criterion. Only about 20 percent qualify as most needy under both criteria. More than half of the high POPPC counties have populations of less than 10,000 people, and almost half are located in the north central and western regions of the country. In contrast, less than a quarter of the high deaths-averted counties have populations of less than 10,000 people, and only 15 percent are in the north central and western regions. More than 80 percent, however, are in the South.

A principal reason for the divergence between the two criteria seems to be that the population-per-physician ratio is not very closely associated with either the need for health care or the use of medical care services. This can be shown by computing the correlation between POPPC and the mortality rate, an indicator of the need for health care, and Medicare expenditures per enrollee, an indicator of the use of medical care. (Direct measures of per capita medical care consumption by age, sex, and race are not available for small geographic areas. Thus, it is necessary to assume that variations across areas in Medicare expenditures per enrollee reflect variation in the per capita medical care consumption of other age groups. Indirect tests of this assumption indicate that it is quite reasonable.) In both cases, the correlation is negative and small in value ($\rho = -0.08$ and -0.18, respectively).

These comparisons suggest that some measure of the use of medical care relative to the need for care may be a better criterion for designating medically underserved counties than a criterion based on the population-per-physician ratio. One possible indicator which is readily available on an annual basis for all counties is the ratio of Medicare expenditures per enrollee to the mortality rate. As noted, the former is a proxy for the use of services and the latter a proxy for the need for services. This ratio is directly related to the deaths-averted criterion, since it can be derived from the same mathematical formula. As a result, the ratio of Medicare expenditures per enrollee to the mortality rate has a large negative correlation with the number of deaths averted per $100,000 increases in medical care expenditures ($\rho = -0.82$). In other words, the number of deaths which would be averted by increasing medical care spending is relatively smaller in counties where the use of services is relatively high compared to the need for services.

The second policy analysis focuses on the need for additional physicians. Since need can only be defined relative to some goal, the analysis assumes an objective of reducing above-average mortality rates in each county and cohort to the national average mortality rate for each cohort in 1970. In effect, the goal of this type of policy is to achieve a specified health improvement regardless of the cost of the policy. The cost of the policy, however, changes dramatically if current physicians can be reallocated costlessly, as opposed to simply adding more physicians to counties where they are needed. However, these two approaches are not identical, since the first in effect equalizes mortality rates across counties, while the second lowers the national mortality rate. (The conversion from increased medical care spending to increased numbers of physicians is based on the estimated relationship across counties between total expenditures for medical care and the total number of active, nonfederal, patient care physicians.)

The analysis suggests that only about 12,000 additional physicians (5 percent of the 1970 total of just under 250,000 active, nonfederal, patient care physicians) would be needed under the costless reallocation scheme. In effect, many physicians would be relocated from low mortality rate counties to high mortality rate counties. In contrast, more than 11 times as many new physicians, about 137,000, would be needed under a policy permitting only net additions to each county. Eighty-two percent of counties would receive some additional physicians under the second approach.

This estimate of additional need seems quite high relative to the 1970 stock of physicians. It is interesting to note, however, that over the last 10 years the number of active patient care physicians has increased by almost this amount. There were about 100,000 more physicians practicing in 1979 than in 1970. Applying the parameters of the health production function to this change in the supply of physicians and, by extension, medical care expenditures per capita suggests that expanded medical care consumption may be responsible for about 20 percent of the decrease in the national mortality rate over this period. Thus, while expanding physician supply by this amount is obviously an expensive policy, it is not one without any benefits.

The estimated percentage change in a county's supply of physicians is strongly related to the mortality rate, the use-need ratio defined previously, and the estimated number of deaths averted for a given increase in medical care spending. Under both allocation schemes, most of the additional physicians are allocated to counties with the largest populations. Counties which lose physicians tend to be smaller counties in SMSAs. Nonmetropolitan counties, particularly those in the smallest population categories, are largely unaffected.

The simulations also suggest that additional physicians would be added primarily to the northeast and north central regions. This contrasts to the regional implications of identifying shortage areas on the basis of the number of deaths averted, which provides additional resources primarily to the South. This difference is apparently because the underlying policies have different objectives. One attempts to maximize the number of deaths averted, given a fixed budget. The other sets a mortality rate reduction as its target, regardless of the cost of the policy.

The third policy analysis explores what is perhaps the most fundamental question of all: how does expanding medical care use compare to other possible policies for reducing mortality rates (improving health)? In effect, this is another way of asking whether medical care's impact on health is large or small in relative terms. Existing data are inadequate to answer this question precisely. But with a number of strong assumptions, it is possible to make an exploratory effort to address this question by computing the cost per death averted for three alternative policies: increasing medical care expenditures by 10 percent; reducing per capita cigarette consumption by 10 percent; and increasing total income by 10 percent for families and unrelated individuals with total money incomes less than $10,000 in 1970. The estimates of the cost of averting a death differ by several orders of magnitude for the three policies. Although the specific values of the estimates are not likely to be highly reliable because of data problems, it appears that an ordinal ranking would probably not be altered if the costs were recomputed with better data or under different assumptions. In particular, the calculations imply that reducing cigarette consumption is the most efficient policy of the three, followed by increasing medical care consumption, and increasing incomes of lower-income persons.

In reporting these various policy implications, it must be emphasized that their primary goal is to illustrate the usefulness of the health production function for evaluating policy issues. The specific implications should not necessarily be applied to current policy problems. The data used by this study are now more than 10 years old and may not accurately reflect current conditions. What these three policy simulations do suggest for current use is that (1) the ratio of population to physicians may not be a very good criterion for identifying areas which need more medical care; (2) the ratio of Medicare expenditures per enrollee to the mortality rate appears to be a much better indicator of underservice; (3) this ratio would probably be even more useful if Medicare expenditures were available by sex and race; and (4) data on expenditures per capita for other population cohorts would also be very useful.

2

THE THEORY OF HEALTH
AND HEALTH PRODUCTION

An important first step toward understanding the relationship between health and medical care is a theoretical model which identifies both
the factors that influence health and the interactions among those factors.
Several global theories have been formulated at a very general level.[1] These
models attempt to group all potential health determinants into a small
number of comprehensive categories, such as environment, behavior, heredity, medical care, and socioeconomic status. Global models represent a
useful starting point but fall short because of their lack of analytic content. The most such models can usually offer is a diagrammatic represen-
tation of the flow of causation. (Figure 1 illustrates two examples.)

To obtain a clearer picture of the structure underlying the health production function, we develop a more formal model based on Grossman's
theory of the demand for health.[2] His approach begins with basic utility
theory and derives relationships for both the demand for health and the
demand for medical care. Health production is then shown to be the process of combining medical care and other goods, given the individual's
efficiency as a health producer and other technical constraints, in order to
attain a desired health stock in each period of time. The advantage of
Grossman's model is that it relates health production to both the demand
for health and the market for medical care. These relationships, in turn,
have important econometric implications.

Global Theories of Health

Most analyses of health, health indicators, or disease patterns begin
with an allusion to the theory of health. Most formulations of the theory of

15

FIGURE 1

Global Health Models

A. Inputs to Health

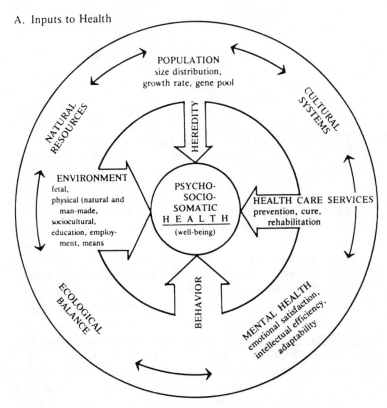

B. Path Analysis of Air Pollution—Mortality Rate Model

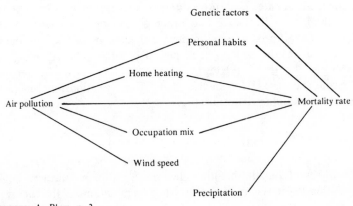

Sources: A. Blum, p. 3.
B. Lave and Seskin, p. 11.

health tend to be categorization schemes which, as indicated by the following excerpts, often provide an opportunity to discuss the relative importance of different factors thought to influence health. A good example of this approach is Blum's four-category model of the inputs to health.[3]

1. Environment

Social, cultural, political, educational, economic, and physical environments all need to be considered here.... Deprivation, frequently in all of these spheres, is the lot of a significant proportion of our citizenry, and its relationship to deficiencies in all kinds of well-being is readily observable. The effects of density on survival and mental illness are not always clear, but the effects of education and to a lesser degree, those of income are clearly health correlated. Vast health improvements and fantastically increased survival rates have been made solely through changes in the physical environment (insect, waste, and water control), with or without significant individual participation. In fact, we have helped to create a world population crisis by this one sided environmental manipulation....

2. Behavior

Personal behavior and habits are major influences on our well-being and our survival (consider smoking, drinking, dangerous driving, overeating, neglect of personal hygiene, delay in seeking medical care, etc.). Their influences can be visualized as the incorporation of prior environmental influences into the makeup of each individual. Whether he has acquired his habit patterns from his parents, his peers, his teachers, or from mass media or advertising, his behavior reflects the way in which he reacts to environmental influences. The actual availability of health services might also be listed among these habit-shaping factors.

3. Heredity

Adverse genetic constitution (which may be confused with deleterious in-utero environmental influences) makes up another major determinant of well-being capacity. Effects of heredity can be modified primarily through applications by the health services of genetic studies and counseling. The in-utero effects of the environment will be avoided through environmental control and health services. The possibilities for confusing effects of heredity and environment after birth have been the subject of many studies....

4. Health Care Services

Undoubtedly a significant factor in overcoming or avoiding illness, disability, and death, health care services nevertheless cannot continue to dominate our perception of how man stays healthy. Planning

for health will involve altering each of the above listed inputs, not just
the traditionally emphasized health (illness) care services. Increasing
the health care input is not the only way, or necessarily the most eco-
nomical or socially intelligent way, to remedy a situation where many
influences are increasing the level of need. Finding other solutions to
the problem may lessen the urgency for application of health care
that often comes too late to avert serious disability or death. Witness
auto accidents caused by defective cars or highways, malaria caused
by uncontrolled mosquitoes, tuberculosis spread in the circumstances
of poverty.

Manipulating inputs to attain a desired end is a complicated affair.
Presumably, removing the financial barriers to medical care, which
can be described either as a removal of an environmental obstacle or
as the extension of accessibility of health services, would result in
some improvements. Yet there is evidence that the differences in
perinatal mortality among the various socioeconomic classes persisted for years in England, despite changes which equalize the availability of services. Differences in relative availability, and variations in
patterns of utilization, persisted even with almost total eligibility for
care.

Lave and Seskin offer a similar (and somewhat more objective) list of
factors affecting mortality. They recognize the arbitrary grouping of factors into the categories of physical characteristics of the population, socioeconomic characteristics, environmental characteristics, and personal characteristics. As table 2 shows, they include medical care consumption in
the last category. Given the specific objective of their research, measuring
the impact of air pollution on mortality, they correctly point out that their
main problem is to control for those factors correlated with air pollution.
In other words, it is not essential to measure and control for *all* factors affecting mortality in order to obtain unbiased statistical estimates of the effects of air pollution.[4]

A more detailed specification of the individual factors which should be
included in each category can be developed from a review of the extensive
literature on geographic variations in mortality rates. (See chapter 3 for a
partial literature review.) Such a listing will be reported in the section on
empirical specification.

An Analytic Theory of Health Production

The theory of health production which underlies this study is based on
Grossman's pathbreaking work on the theories of the demands for health

TABLE 2

FACTORS AFFECTING MORTALITY

PHYSICAL	SOCIOECONOMIC	ENVIRONMENTAL	PERSONAL
Age distribution	Income distribution	Air pollution levels	Smoking habits
Sex distribution	Occupation mix	Radiation levels	Medical care (quality and quantity)
Race distribution	Housing density or crowding	Climatological characteristics	Exercise habits
	Differential migration	Domestic factors (home-heating equipment,	Nutritional history
		heating fuels, etc.)	Genetic effects

SOURCE: Lave and Seskin, p. 10.

and medical care. His model begins with the assumption of an intertemporal utility function with health and other goods as arguments. (The utility function is a concept used to summarize the value that people derive from various goods and activities). For the sake of simplicity, we focus on only a single time period and also ignore issues associated with the allocation of time among different activities (producing health, producing other consumption goods, work, leisure, and illness). Therefore, utility is simply a function of the stock of health, H, and other consumption goods.

The quantity of health attained in a particular period is the result of combining medical care, M, and own time, T. Other factors, however, clearly affect a person's efficiency as a health producer. In other words, the actual amount of health produced for a given combination of M and T will also depend on the person's initial health level, education, marital status, characteristics of the environment, cigarette consumption, alcohol consumption, exercise, diet, and income. Variations or changes in these factors will shift the location of the health production function.

The production relationship between health and medical care is plotted in quadrant 2 of figure 2. (All axes measures positive quantities in this figure). As the quantity of medical care used is increased, holding other factors constant, the amount of health produced increases. At some point, of course, additional medical care use may not produce any additional health, that is, the curve in quadrant 2 may become vertical beyond some value of M. An increase in the value of an efficiency-reducing factor, say cig-

FIGURE 2

THE DEMAND FOR HEALTH, HEALTH PRODUCTION, AND THE MARKET FOR MEDICAL CARE

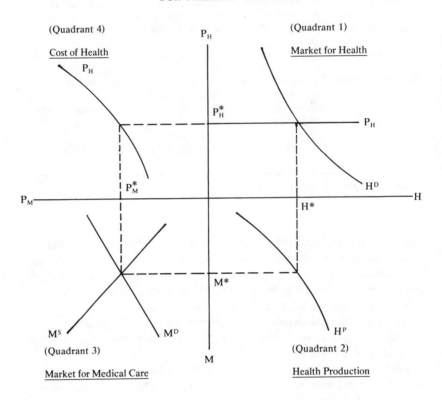

Key: P_H = Price of health.
     H = Quantity of health.
     M = Quantity of medical care.
     P_M = Price of medical care.
     H^D = Health demand function.
     H^P = Health production function.
     M^S = Supply of medical care.
     M^D = Demand for medical care.

arette smoking, will shift the entire function down and to the left. In effect, less health is produced for a given quantity of medical care consumption.

Grossman shows that the amount of health desired depends on its value relative to that of other goods, the cost of producing health, and the person's command over resources (wealth).[5] The key feature of the resulting demand function for health, which is shown in quadrant 1 of figure 2, is that an increase in the cost of producing health, P_H, lowers the level of health chosen. Factors which shift the location of the entire function affect the quantity of health demanded for a given value of P_H. For example, a change in a factor which affects the value of healthy time, such as the wage rate, will shift the demand for health. As a result, people in high wage occupations will demand more health for a given value of P_H than people in low wage occupations, other things being equal.

The demand function for health shows the amount of health stock which would be demanded at various values of P_H. The actual quantity desired depends on the value of P_H faced by the individual. Since P_H is defined to be the cost of increasing the stock of health by one unit, it depends on the costs of increasing the quantities of the inputs in the health production function. In particular, P_H will be positively related to the price of medical care, P_M, and the price of time, W, which can also be thought of as the wage rate. (P_H would also be affected by the cost of changing other factors which influence the health production function. For example, time spent exercising may increase health production efficiency but also increases the cost of health.) Quadrant 4 of figure 2 illustrates the relationship between P_H and P_M.

An increase in any of the other cost-increasing factors, such as W, would shift the cost function upwards. Note, however, that P_H is assumed to be independent of the stock of health, H.[6] Thus in quadrant 1, P_H is simply a horizontal line. The intersection of P_H with the demand-for-health function determines the desired health stock.

One feature of this model is that it shows how the demand for health and the health production relationship in quadrants 1 and 2 help to determine the demand for medical care, that is, the relationship between medical care use and the price of medical care. The demand function for medical care, noted by M^D in quadrant 3 of figure 2, postulates that the quantity of care demanded increases as the price of medical care decreases. Suppose that the demand for health increases, that is, the entire H^D function in quadrant 1 shifts to the right. (This might happen if an increase in wages increased the demand for healthy work days). Other things held constant, the shift in H^D would increase the quantity of medical care required to attain the new equilibrium level of H. The impact on the market for medical care would be to shift the M^D function down and to the left—more medical care would be demanded at every value of P_M.

As another example, the onset of an epidemic could be thought of as a reduction in production efficiency, that is, the health production function shifts down and to the left. If medical care use is not increased, then the amount of health produced would be less than the amount desired, H*. In order to return to the desired health level, medical care use increases. As the epidemic subsides, possibly because of the increase in medical care use, the efficiency of the production process increases so that the production function, the consumption of medical care, and the level of health return to their initial levels. In effect, this example illustrates the well-known proposition that sicker people will generally use more medical care.

Finally, the model is completed by postulating a supply-of-medical-care function, noted by M^S in quadrant 3. This shows how differences in the supply of medical care can influence the level of health by affecting the cost of producing a unit of health. Thus, for example, an expansion in the supply of medical care, other things unchanged, should lower the price of medical care, P_M, which in turn leads to a lower cost of producing health, P_H. At a lower value of P_H, more health will be demanded, thus absorbing the expanded supply of medical care.

Although this approach to developing a theory of health may seem somewhat cumbersome, it has several advantages over the global approach described earlier. First, the simultaneous relationship between the production of health and the quantity of medical care demanded is clearly established. Medical care use influences the level of health, but health also helps to determine the quantity of care demanded. Second, the model relates the market for medical care to health production. This is important because it links variables from the market for medical care with the health production process. Finally, the model can generate hypotheses and identify potentially offsetting effects among the complex interrelationships. These capabilities are important as guides for specifying the empirical analysis and interpreting its results.

One should also note that the model represented by figure 2 is really quite consistent with the global theories of health alluded to earlier. In particular, behavioral factors affect the locations of both the demand for health and health production functions and, consequently, the demand for medical care as well. Environmental and biological factors influence the efficiency of health production. Thus, for example, older people are probably less efficient producers of health than younger people because of natural biological deterioration with age. Therefore, even though medical care use increases with age, health levels will be lower because of reduced production efficiency. Finally, changes in the market for medical care can also be related to the level of health through the effects on the cost of producing health. In sum, the two approaches include the same types of variables. However, the second is a much better guide for empirical specification of the health production relationship.

3

VARIATIONS IN MORTALITY RATES—A
SELECTED LITERATURE REVIEW

This chapter provides a selected summary and review of the extensive literature on factors associated with variations in mortality rates. The first section focuses on studies of adult and age-adjusted mortality rates, and the second reviews analyses of infant mortality rates. Within each of these groups, the prior research is subdivided, primarily on the basis of methodological approach. The first, and far more extensive group, will be referred to as epidemiologically oriented. By and large, these studies emphasize the identification of differences in mortality rates for various population groups classified by one or more of the following criteria: place of residence, city or county population, age, sex, race, nativity, social class, marital status, parity, education, income, occupation, and cause of death. Less emphasis is placed upon explaining observed variations and, consequently, analytic methods are usually limited to simple and partial correlation analysis and occasionally, simple regression analysis.

This literature is fairly well known and has been thoroughly summarized in several other sources.[1] In addition, it has not focused primarily on the question of the marginal effect of medical care on reductions in mortality. Therefore, its main contribution to this study is to suggest potential independent variables which ought to be controlled for in order to attain unbiased estimates of the effect of medical care on mortality rates.

Of more direct relevance to this project is the small number of studies, primarily by economists, that have attempted to specify and estimate formal models explaining variations in mortality rates. These analyses share the health production function framework and provide the theoretical and methodological backgrounds for this study.

23

ADULT AND AGE-ADJUSTED MORTALITY RATES

1. THE EPIDEMIOLOGICAL LITERATURE

The first thing to be gleaned from the epidemiological literature is that significant variations in mortality rates do in fact exist for all levels of geographic classification: census regions, census divisions, states, economic subregions, SMSAs, and census tracts within cities. These results continue to hold when crude mortality data are adjusted for variations in age distributions and broken down by sex and race.[2] Most of the studies that will be mentioned here have attempted to explore one or more factors thought to be related to geographic variations in mortality rates. For the sake of convenience, relevant findings will be grouped according to whether a variable measures a population characteristic or an environmental characteristic.

Perhaps the most commonly used variables have been proxies for socioeconomic status, for example, per capita income, median family income, condition of housing, or occupation. Looking at the historical record and using crude measures of social class such as noble/nonnoble birth, taxpayer/nontaxpayer, or laborer/nonlaborer, Antonovsky found a consistent inverse relationship between mortality and social class.[3] Interestingly, he also observed that over time the mortality gradient between classes has diminished. Altenderfer found a similar relationship between mortality and per capita income for 92 cities over 1939–1940, as did Woolsey for a select sample of low mortality rural counties in the west north central region.[4] Kitagawa and Hauser reported negative correlations between median family income and age-adjusted mortality for samples of Chicago census tracts for 1950.[5] The results held for both sexes in both predominantly white and predominantly black tracts. At the same time, the percentage of dwelling units in substandard condition had a consistently positive correlation. However, for 201 SMSAs over 1959–1961, the simple correlation between median family income and age-adjusted mortality was negative for nonwhite males ($-.296$) and females ($-.402$), but positive, though small for white males ($.053$) and females ($.098$). A similar pattern was observed for states.

The positive signs for whites' incomes appear to be consistent with the hypothesis that the beneficial effects of increased income (living standards) on mortality may have an upper limit which may already have been attained, on average, by certain population subgroups.[6] (This issue was explored at greater length by Auster et al. and Silver and will be discussed.[7])

Other attempts to explain geographic variations in mortality rates have looked at the degree of urbanization as a potential causal factor. Sauer and Donnel analyzed mortalilty rates for white males, ages 45 to 64, over the period 1959–1961 for 231 state economic areas with fewer than 5 percent nonwhite population.[8] Simple correlations were computed between a number of variables and mortality from all causes, from cardiovascular diseases, from coronary diseases, and from malignant neoplasms except lung. The variables with the highest correlations were percentage rural farm population ($-.45$ to $-.65$), percentage females employed (.51 to .61), and percentage of men over age 65 who are working ($-.08$ to $-.34$).

The last variable is probably a crude proxy for average health levels, since it seems likely that at older ages health is a major determinant of labor force status. The negative correlation with degree of rurality is consistent with several other studies which have found an inverse relation between rurality and mortality.[9] Explanations of this finding have speculated that urban residents face greater risks of death from infectious diseases, air pollution, and violence. The positive correlations with the percentage of females employed may reflect the correlations between female labor force participation and both widowhood and low family income.

Another variable found to be inversely related to mortality is education. Kitagawa and Hauser found that differentials in age-adjusted mortality rates were greater for women than for men in 1960, and that the size of the differential varied with age for men: there was practically no difference in mortality rates for men above the age of 65.[10] When the separate effect of income was controlled through stratification, education still had an inverse relationship, but the size of the differential was reduced. For example, in a comparison between white males, 25 to 64 years old, with less than 8 years of education and those with more than 16 years of education, the mortality differential was reduced from 40 to 21 percent when income was held constant. Studies of individuals' health levels by Grossman and Manheim have demonstrated that schooling has a positive effect on health, independent of income and other factors.[11]

Marital status has been cited by Fuchs, Orcutt et al., and Sheps as influencing mortality.[12] Using 1948–1951 data, Sheps found that married people generally had the lowest mortality rate within age-color-sex stratified cells. It has been hypothesized that this may be due to self-selection, since people with health problems are probably less likely to marry, and to the caring activities provided by a spouse. The latter effect seems to be greater for males than females, on the basis of a larger married/unmarried differential for males. Additionally, widowed and divorced people had higher mortality rates than either single (never married) or married people. Orcutt et al. obtained very similar results using multivariate regression methods on age-sex-race-specific county group data for 1970.

The positive relationship between smoking and morbidity and mortality at the individual level is now well known. Friedman analyzed the effect of smoking on health using state cross-sectional data for 1960.[13] Estimates of per capita cigarette consumption were generated from tax data collected by the National Tobacco Tax Association. The simple correlation between the age-adjusted mortality rate for coronary heart disease and per capita cigarette consumption was .55. Using 1950 data for 33 states, the correlation was .63 for deaths from coronary heart disease for white males, 25 to 64 years old, and .81 for deaths from lung cancer. Partial correlations controlling for urbanization and water hardness were also significantly positive.

Also well known is the fact that blacks of both sexes tend to have higher age-specific mortality rates than whites, controlling for both geographic region and population size.[14] Most authors feel that these results reflect the cumulative and pervasive effects of lower incomes, living standards, and education levels experienced by blacks. In addition to variations by race, nativity also appears to be related to differences in mortality rates. Kitagawa and Hauser, and Sauer found that foreign-born U.S. residents tended to have higher mortality rates than the native-born population (excluding American Indians).[15] However, within the foreign-born, those from Japan and northwest Europe seem to have mortality rates lower than the U.S. average.[16] It has been hypothesized that these types of variations are due to the combined effects of genetic, dietary, and cultural differences. However, the identification of specific causal agents and mechanisms at the individual level has not yet advanced sufficiently to explain fully the aggregate correlations.

Turning to studies which have examined the effects of environmental variables, Schroeder computed simple correlations between a number of characteristics of water supply and various mortality rates for the 1949-1951 period.[17] His most consistent finding was a negative correlation between mortality and water hardness. For white males, 45 to 64 years old, across 163 metropolitan areas, the correlation was −.33 for all causes. At the state level, correlations of −.38, −.55, and −.10 were found for mortality from all causes, cardiovascular diseases, and noncardiovascular diseases, respectively.

Sauer and Donnel computed correlations between a variety of variables and cause-specific mortality rates for 126 metropolitan areas over 1959-1961.[18] The largest correlations in absolute value were for two measures of climate, annual precipitation and average daily January temperature change, and for elevation above sea level. States examined the relationships between daily mortality over a four-year period in Birmingham, Alabama and a number of weather variables.[19] Using multiple correlation techniques, he found a significant relationship between weather and daily total mortality. This relationship was larger for the elderly and for whites than for others. Among various causes of death the relationship was strongest for circulatory and respiratory causes but relatively weak for cancers and accidental causes.

Lave and Seskin investigated the association between total, infant, and disease-specific mortality and a variety of measures of air pollution for 117 SMSAs in 1960 and 1961.[20] They estimated a series of linear regression equations with measures of particles and sulphates in the air and several sociodemographic characteristics as independent variables. Several of the air pollution variables were statistically significant in the various regressions and all had positive signs. For total deaths, for example, a 10 percent reduction in mean particles per cubic meter was estimated to have the effect of reducing the total mortality rate by .53 percent.

In sum, these studies have suggested a number of variables which ought to be included as control factors in any attempt to estimate a mortality production function. Mortality rates were shown to vary by age, sex, race, income levels, urbanization, marital status, occupation, education, cigarette consumption, nativity, water hardness, air pollution, and climate. Since most of these studies used only simple analytic techniques, one cannot readily infer what the marginal contribution may be of any of these factors to changes in mortality, nor can one be confident that they will necessarily maintain their apparent significance when analyzed in a multivariate context. Consequently the primary role of this literature is to suggest variables which ought to be considered in specifying the health production function.

2. THE ECONOMICS LITERATURE

Building upon earlier observations of Fuchs on the role of health and the costs of mortality to the United States economy, Auster et al. set out to investigate the basic question which underlies this study: "What is the contribution of medical services as opposed to environmental factors to changes in the health of the population?"[21] They also noted the need to identify "... the contribution of each of the factors of production which combine to produce medical services."

Their model postulated a multiplicative relationship between the age-sex-adjusted death rate, measures of medical care consumption, and a number of environmental variables included as controls for variations in population and geographic area characteristics. (The unit of analysis was the state and all data were for 1960.) The environmental variables included percentage nonwhite, income, education, percentage of population in SMSAs, percentage employed in manufacturing, percentage in white-collar occupations, alcohol and cigarette consumption per capita, percentage of females not in the labor force, and the presence of a medical school in the state.

Specifically, the functional form they used can be represented by

$$H = C_1 M^{\sigma_0} \prod_{i=1}^{n} X^{\sigma_i} e^{\epsilon_1} \qquad\qquad (3.1)$$

where H is a health indicator, C_1 is a constant, M is the measure of medical care consumption, the X_i are the other independent variables, and ϵ_1 is a random error. The elasticity of mortality with respect to medical care, σ_0 is the primary parameter of interest. (Elasticity is defined here as the percentage change in the mortality rate which would result from a 1 percent change in the consumption of medical care.) Two approaches were taken to the measurement of M. One was to substitute medical care expenditures per capita directly into equation (3.1). The second approach postulated a second multiplicative production function for medical care services,

$$M = C_2 \prod_{j=1}^{k} Z_j^{\gamma_j} e^{\epsilon_2} \qquad\qquad (3.2)$$

where the Z_j are measures of stocks of medical care resources, such as physicians and hospital beds per capita. The right-hand side of equation (3.2) was then substituted directly into equation (3.1).[22]

The model was estimated by both ordinary (OLS) and two-stage least squares (TSLS) regression analysis and in both linear and log-linear forms. Use of TSLS was justified by the argument that the consumption of medical care services is jointly determined with mortality rates. Initially, death rates for whites and nonwhites were combined and the percentage black population used as an independent variable. However, this variable was highly correlated with some of the other variables. As a result, parameter estimates were unreliable. Therefore, they based their remaining estimations on data for whites only, although no adjustment was made to the medical care variables.[23]

Using a variety of specifications, they concluded that a 1 percent increase in the quantity of medical services is associated with approximately a .1 percent decrease in white, age-sex-adjusted mortality. Environmental factors, particularly income and education, had a larger quantitative impact on mortality. Education had a negative effect, as expected, but the coefficient of income was positive. The authors speculated that above some point, rising income may be associated with occupational conditions (such as stress, lack of exercise) and behavior changes (such as in diet, increased auto travel) which have adverse effects on mortality. Urbanization was not significant, but the labor force variables, percentage in manufacturing and percentage of females not in the labor force, were positive and negative, respectively. The positive relationship between smoking and mortality was confirmed. Finally, states with medical schools had slightly lower mortality rates than those without.

An interesting implication derived from their estimates was an explanation of the paradox that the age-adjusted death rate had not declined appreciably between 1955 and 1965 even though there had been a substantial increase in medical care consumption per capita. Very simply, their coefficients implied that increases in medical care consumption and education should have reduced mortality by about 7 percent. However, this expected decrease was roughly offset due to rising incomes and cigarette consumption.

Although this study must be considered an important contribution to efforts to explain the effects of medical care on mortality, it did have several shortcomings. First, as pointed out by the authors, it would have been preferable to estimate separate age-sex-race-specific production functions, since, as indicated by the earlier literature, there may be important differences in the factors affecting specific mortality rates. A second problem is the use of the state as the unit of analysis. While this choice is frequently necessitated by the lack of required data for smaller geographic units, it is likely that much intrastate heterogeneity is masked by the use of state averages. Finally, although the inability to adjust the medical consumption variables may not be too costly when dealing with the white population, this may be more problematic in estimating production functions for more narrowly defined mortality rates.

Silver extended the work by Auster et al. in essentially two ways [24] First, the mortality data were disaggregated by race and sex, and second, relationships were estimated for SMSAs as well as states. This study, however, was concerned less with assessing the effect of medical care on mortality than with untangling the influences of income, education, and a variety of other variables on race- and sex-specific mortality rates. Silver based the specification of his empirical model on an appeal to the " ... 'consumer demand function for health' and other variables. The variables in the demand function are further classified as economic, informational, or taste."[25] The initial formulation included variables such as alternative measures of the command over resources (total family income, total individual income, labor and nonlabor income), health information (education), taste measures (marital status, fertility, region), and other factors (size of residence, percentage black population, the ulcer death rate as a proxy for psychological pressures, cigarette consumption, climate, air pollution, and physicians per capita as a proxy for medical care availability).

Although Silver approached the problem from a different vantage than Auster et al., his empirical method was very similar. He used ordinary (OLS) and two-stage least squares (TSLS) regression analysis to estimate the parameters of linear and log-linear specifications of the relationships between various mortality rates and variables measuring a variety of medical care, economic, and environmental factors.

In general, the results did not tend to support the earlier findings of a positive relationship between household income and mortality (although the state estimate for white males was positive). However, this conclusion was derived from a regression which excluded measures of schooling, physicians per capita, and fertility on the grounds of multicollinearity. When income was divided into its labor and nonlabor components, the effect of labor income tended to be positive (or less negative) while the coefficient of nonlabor income was consistently negative. The positive effect of labor income was strongest for white males, which suggests that for this subset of the population the factors associated with increasing income may have deleterious side effects.

The only medical care variable included in the regressions was physicians per capita. Its coefficient was negative and significant in the OLS-SMSA estimations for white females and black males and females. The coefficients were insignificant with mixed signs in the state equations and in the TSLS-SMSA equations. The result for the state equation for white males was a negative, though small and insignificant coefficient, which is consistent with the Auster et al. finding. The only significant negative state coefficients were in the black female equations. The elasticities were $-.15$ and $-.18$.

Finally, several additional variables were introduced in the attempt to measure health information, variations in tastes, and living standards. The percentage of the population married had a generally negative and significant coefficient, and the fertility rate and the ulcer-related death rates were both generally significant and positive. The schooling variable was consistently negative, as predicted, and frequently significant. This suggests the importance of health information on the health process. Cigarette consumption was consistently positive and significant, supporting the earlier findings of Auster et al. and Friedman.[26] Per capita welfare payments had a negative effect on mortality, and they were statistically significant in the female regressions, reflecting the probably greater dependence of women on welfare support. Of the climate and air pollution variables, average annual temperature was consistently negative and significant in all but the equation for black males; results for the air pollution variables were mixed, although a measure of sulphur dioxide density seemed most promising.

In general, disaggregating the mortality data by race and sex revealed that factors affecting mortality have differential impacts on different subpopulations. This was particularly true for income, which had a negative and quantitatively greater impact on black mortality than on white mortality. In the SMSA equations, physicians per capita also had a larger effect on black mortality than on white mortality.

A paper by Margaret Reid focused more closely on the somewhat surprising result of some of these state-level econometric studies that current income was positively related to age-adjusted mortality rates for white males in 1960.[27] Primary emphasis was given to the importance of age as a determinant of mortality risk and the complex interactions among age, health, education, income, and migration. In addition, she explored potential biases arising from the use of state level data and from census undercounting of state populations. (The latter are the denominators used in computing state mortality rates.)

The major thrust of her critique is that the econometric analyses do not adequately take account of the impact of age on the independent variables in their statistical models. Her implicit model asserts that genetic endowment and the cumulative influence of factors affecting physiological changes are the principal determinants of what she calls the stock of health (HST). As one ages, HST becomes less and less subject to the influence of current consumption activities, and more and more determined by prior experience. Since, in general, we cannot directly observe HST, age is its best available indirect measure. This is reflected in the substantial increase in mortality rates with age (excepting infant mortality).

Within a state, the age distribution of the population also affects average levels of income, education, and migration. The reasons for this are fairly straightforward and can be summarized as follows:

    a. Current money income depends primarily on the average hourly (weekly) wage and the amount of time worked. In the early stages of the life cycle, wages tend to be low. Income rises as wages increase with experience, career advancement, etc. Finally, at retirement reported income falls sharply as hours worked are drastically reduced. Thus, income will on average exhibit an inverted U-shaped relationship with age.

b. Average education levels decline with age primarily because of secular changes in access to public education and in the demands for an educated labor force.

c. Population mobility is generally higher for both the young and the healthy. This suggests that migration patterns affect the distribution of health stock both directly (by increasing the supply of healthy people in states with positive rates of net migration) and indirectly (by increasing the proportion of the population at young ages).[28]

How do the econometric studies reviewed by Reid deal with these problems? The impact of age on mortality is generally acknowledged and accounted for by constructing an age-adjusted mortality rate for use as the dependent variable. The usual approach taken is to apply age-specific mortality rates for each state to some reference age distribution, usually that of the entire United States. One property of the resultant age-adjusted mortality rate is that it is quite sensitive to variations in mortality for older age groups. The correlations between the age-adjusted mortality rate for white males across states in 1960 and age-specific rates for the 55–64 and 65–74 age groups are .881 and .913, respectively.[29]

None of the studies she examined, however, explicitly accounted for the effect of age distribution on average levels of education and income. Furthermore, the studies did not generally attempt to control for the effects of migration patterns or possible census undercounting. Given the problems of multicollinearity and lack of variation inherent in state level data, as well as the measurement errors just discussed, Reid argues that there is good reason to believe that the reported results are subject to bias.

Given these problems, what changes could one make to improve the reliability of the statistical estimates? First, as Reid explicitly suggested, analysis of age-specific (and by implication sex- and race-specific) mortality rates is preferable.[30] This is likely to reduce the correlation between income and education, which depends strongly on age. Furthermore, the effect of the health stock, which is largely unobservable, is more likely to be held constant when age is held fixed. Second, one should try to limit analyses to geographic areas which are reasonably homogenous with respect to market conditions and unspecified factors. At the state level, stratification is limited by the number of observations and, for some variables, the relatively small range of natural variation. Third, key independent variables, particularly education, types of income, and family structure, should be constructed to match the population underlying the mortality rate being analyzed.

The recent study by Orcutt et al. serves to illustrate these advantages.[31] They estimated several statistical relationships at the county group level between age-sex-race-specific mortality rates and a number of independent variables drawn from the public use sample of the 1970 Census. In 12 to 14 equations, education and income had the expected negative signs, and in the two cases where the signs were positive they were not statistically significant.[32]

Infant Mortality

Infant mortality refers to deaths occuring between the 1st and 364th day of life. However, the risks and causes of death vary dramatically with age over this period. For example, the number of deaths per 1000 live births is approximately 20 times higher at the end of the first day of life than at the end of the first week of life.[33] By the second half of the first year, the mortality rate drops to 0.4 per 1,000 live births, compared to 16.1 in the first month.[34] Deaths in the earliest stage of life are most frequently caused by immaturity, postnatal asphyxia and atelectasis, birth injuries, and congenital malformations. In later periods the most common causes are infectious diseases and accidents. Because of these differences, infant mortality is frequently divided into two classes: neonatal deaths, which occur between 1 and 27 days, and postneonatal deaths, which occur between 28 and 364 days after birth. Finally, a third category of infant deaths comprises those which take place in utero, that is, fetal deaths. Since the causes and factors associated with fetal deaths are sometimes thought to be very similar to those associated with neonatal deaths, the two are often combined into a single category called perinatal mortality, which includes fetal deaths of more than 20 weeks gestation and neonatal deaths. Table 3 summarizes these definitions.

Studies of infant deaths frequently distinguish between two classes of factors, biologic and socioeconomic, thought to be related to variations in mortality rates. Among the former are birth weight, gestation period, maternal age, birth order, race, sex, and previous pregnancy outcome. The latter usually include family income, education, occupation, marital status, and the use of medical care. The literature is nearly unanimous with regard to the relationships between the biologic factors and infant

TABLE 3

DEFINITIONS OF VARIOUS MORTALITY RATES

$$FMR = \frac{\text{fetal deaths}}{\text{fetal deaths} + \text{live births}} = \text{fetal mortality rate}$$

$$NMR = \frac{\text{deaths from 1 to 27 days}}{\text{live births}} = \text{neonatal mortality rate}$$

$$PNMR = \frac{\text{deaths from 28 to 364 days}}{\text{live births}} = \text{postneonatal mortality rate}$$

$$PRMR = FMR + NMR$$
$$= \frac{\text{fetal deaths} + \text{deaths from 1 to 27 days}}{\text{fetal deaths} + \text{live births}} = \text{perinatal mortality rate}$$

$$IMR = NMR + PNMR = \frac{\text{deaths from 1 to 364 days}}{\text{live births}} = \text{infant mortality rate}$$

mortality. Therefore, these findings will be summarized briefly. (For more detailed reviews, see Kessner et al.; Shapiro et al.; and Phillips and Williams.)[35] Results regarding the impact of socioeconomic factors, on the other hand, are much less clearcut. Since this is the arena where public policies are likely to be directed, more detailed attention will be paid to findings in this area.

Almost all studies agree that the single most important factor explaining infant mortality is weight at birth. Data from the 1960 U.S. Live-Birth Cohort study show that the mortality rate for infants weighing less than 2,500 grams, 190.3 deaths per 1,000 live births, is almost 20 times that for infants weighing more than 2,500 grams.[36] Mortality rates decline dramatically with increases in weight, reaching a minimum of 8.0 deaths per 1,000 live births at weights between 3,501 and 4,000 grams.[37] Death rates increase slightly at heavier birth weights.

Gestational age is also generally inversely associated with infant mortality. The infant mortality rate is about 80 times larger at 20 to 27 weeks gestation than at 40 weeks gestation.[38] However, Phillips and Williams have demonstrated that the strength of this relationship operates through the effects of gestational age on birth weight.[39] Birth weight alone explained about 81 percent of the variation in neonatal mortality rates across 159 age-weight-race cells; adding gestational age to their equation explained only an additional 3 percent of the variance.[40]

Maternal age is a third factor correlated with infant mortality rates. More than 50 percent of live births occur to women between the ages of 20 and 29. Infant mortalilty rates in this age category are roughly half those at either extreme of the age distribution (under 15 or over 45 years old).[41] However, only a very small proportion of births occur to women in the two extreme age groups.

Although mortality rates at each stage of infancy have been declining steadily over the last 15 years, rates for nonwhites (primarily blacks) have remained about twice as high as rates for whites. While the factors explaining these differences are undoubtedly complex, part of the explanation seems to lie in the higher proportions of nonwhite infants born at low birth weights, with short gestations, and to very young mothers. (Table 4 illustrates these differences.) As will be discussed further, racial differences in income, education, use of medical care, and general socioeconomic status probably also contribute to observed differences in mortality rates.

The remaining biological factors include sex, birth order, plurality, and prior pregnancy loss. Although the underlying causes of the observed differences in mortality rates are not clear, these patterns are distinct and have persisted over time. In general, female infants have lower mortality rates than male infants; lower birth order is associated with lower mortality rates; single births have a much higher survival probability than plural births; and infants born to women who have not had any prior pregnancy loss have lower mortality rates. Table 5 reports data from various years to illustrate the magnitudes of these differences.

Turning to socioeconomic factors and infant mortality, several studies

TABLE 4

PERCENTAGE OF BIRTHS IN HIGH-RISK CATEGORIES
BY RACE, 1960

	White	Nonwhite
Percentage of births < 2500 grams	6.84	12.95
Percentage of births < 36 weeks gestation	3.16	6.06
Percentage of births to mothers < 20 years old	12.81	20.25
Percentage of births to mothers < 15 years old	0.07	0.65
Percentage of plural births	1.93	2.63

SOURCE: U.S. Department of Health, Education and Welfare, Public Health Service (PHS), National Center for Health Statistics (NCHS), 1960 live-birth cohort, various tables.

TABLE 5

Differences in Various Infant Mortality Rates
By Selected Biological Risk Factors

Risk Factor	Year	Mortality Rate (per 1,000 live births)
Birth order	1964–1966	
First		18.1
Fourth		21.2
Fifth		25.2
Sixth and higher		29.7
Sex	1960	
Female		21.8
Male		28.3
Plurality	1960	
Single		23.3
Plural		116.0
Prior fetal deaths	1964–1966	
None		18.3
One		28.8
Two or more		43.6

Sources: HEW, PHS, NCHS, *Infant Mortality Rates: Relationships with Mother's Reproductive History*, p. 5 (prior fetal deaths) and p. 27 (birth order); and *A Study of Infant Mortality from Linked Records*, p. 30 (sex) and p. 76 (plurality).

have examined alternative proxies for economic status: father's occupation,[42] neighborhood income level,[43] family income,[44] mother's education,[45] and illegitimacy.[46] In general, bivariate comparisons between any of these proxies and various infant mortality rates show an inverse relationship—infant mortality rates decline as socioeconomic status increases. However, when risk factors, especially low birth weight, are taken into account, the mortality differential among socioeconomic classes becomes much smaller and in some cases insignificant.[47] This suggests that the primary influence of socioeconomic status may occur through its impact on risk at birth (low birth weight), rather than as an independent determinant of infant mortality.

Several of these same studies have also examined the impact of various measures of medical care use. Shah and Abbey, Kessner et al., and Erhardt et al. compared infant mortality rates for women who obtained early prenatal care and women who received no prenatal care.[48] Even after adjusting for several possibly confounding variables, the no prenatal care group had higher mortality rates. Jackson and Norris, and Erhardt et al.

compared mortality rates by the type of hospital in which the infant was born.[49] In both studies, infants born in private hospitals had lower mortality rates than infants born in public hospitals. The Jackson and Norris study also found that infants not born in hospitals had higher mortality rates than infants born in hospitals, except for those whose mothers did not receive any known prenatal care.[50] Kessner et al. combined information on the time of the first prenatal visit, the number of prenatal visits, and the type of hospital service (private or general) where delivery took place to group births into three medical care classes: adequate, intermediate, and inadequate.[51] Even after controlling for race, education, and birth risk, mortality rates were lowest among infants whose mothers received adequate medical care.

Probably the most sophisticated approach taken to measuring the impact of medical care while controlling for expected risk is that used by Williams in two recent studies.[52] In both cases, expected risk was measured as a weighted average of the distribution of births by birth weights. The weights were national, weight-specific mortality rates. In effect, he assumed that the impact of both socioeconomic and biological factors operate primarily through the birth-weight distribution. These factors are compressed into a single variable, the expected mortality rate (ED), which is computed as

$$ED_j = \sum_{i=1}^{n} D_i N_{ij}, \tag{3.3}$$

where D_i is the national mortality rate for the ith birth-weight class, and N_{ij} is the fraction of births in the ith birth-weight class in the jth area.

This approach was applied to state data for 1968 to estimate a production function of the same general form used in several studies of adult mortality, that is,

$$D_j = C \cdot ED_j^{\alpha} T_j^{\beta} \qquad j = 1, \ldots, 48 \text{ states.} \tag{3.4}$$

D_j in this study was defined as the neonatal mortality rate, on the grounds that the effects of medical care can be observed within a short time period (75 percent of infant deaths occur during the first month); neonatal mortality occurs with a high frequency; and the group of physicians providing the bulk of care, obstetricians, are readily identifiable. The medical care variable, T, which was defined as obstetricians per 1,000 live births, had an elasticity of $-.097$ (which is very similar to the Auster et al. magnitude) and was statistically significant. The coefficient of the expected mortality rate was positive, significant, and much greater (.862). As Williams pointed out, however, altering the availability of medical care may be more cost-effective than attempting to alter the environment.

In the more recent study, Williams used the same approach to evaluate perinatal medical care delivered in 504 California hospitals.[53] Crude perinatal mortality rates differed sixteenfold across the hospitals in his analysis. After adjusting for expected mortality on the basis of the distribution of newborns by weight at birth, sex, race, and plurality, differences across hospitals were reduced to a factor of two. Subsequent analysis revealed that the ratio of observed to expected perinatal mortality rates "...was significantly lower in larger delivery services, in urban hospitals, in hospitals performing above-average numbers of caesarean sections, in those recording Apgar scores, and in hospitals having higher specialist-to-generalist ratios."[54]

Finally, Grossman and Jacobowitz have focused on the impact of Medicaid policies and the liberalization of abortion laws on race-specific neonatal mortality rates in 1970.[55] Using a series of dummy variables to characterize different states' policies, their preliminary results suggest that liberal coverage of first-time pregnancies by Medicaid has no effect on white neonatal mortality, and a small negative impact on black neonatal mortality. Abortion law liberalization appears to have been the single most important factor contributing to lower neonatal mortality rates for both white and black newborns.

Summary

This literature review had two objectives. One was to identify factors which ought to be included in analyses of geographic variations in adult and infant mortality rates. The second was to set the context for this study in terms of extending the findings of past research. With regard to the first goal, the studies reviewed identified a number of factors which ought to be included in the empirical analysis. Although most of the studies were not carried out within an explicit theory of health, the various factors identified can be readily assigned to the various macrofactors thought to influence health. Specific variables include age, sex, race, economic status, urbanization, marital status, occupation, education, cigarette consumption, nativity, water hardness, air pollution, climate, and risk at birth. Various measures of these factors will be included in the subsequent analysis.

This review also indicated the existing ambiguity and inconsistency regarding the effects of medical care and income on mortality rates.

Studies reporting both positive and negative relationships were cited. However, studies by Auster et al., Williams, and Williams and Phillips, which explicitly incorporated the health production function framework, did report an inverse relationship between mortality rates and medical care use. The magnitude of the relationship was surprisingly similar in these studies—a 10 percent increase in medical care use was associated with approximately a 1 percent decrease in the mortality rate. This is surprising because these studies used different mortality rates: age-adjusted in Auster et al., and infant mortality in the other two, and different measures of medical care: expenditures per capita in the first case and obstetricians per 1,000 live births in the others. These studies, however, did use similar functional forms and empirical methods.

Finally, the review highlighted the lack of analyses of age-sex-race-specific mortality rates and the difficulties of coordinating underlying population bases for measuring both dependent and independent variables. Another shortcoming, particularly of the multivariate studies, has been the lack of analyses using geographic units smaller than the state. Finally, none of the studies has developed policy implications directly relevant to issues of physician distribution and medical care resource allocation. This study will attempt to extend current information along each of these dimensions.

4

DEFINING A HEALTH INDICATOR AND MEASURING MEDICAL CARE USE

The theory outlined in chapter 2 described in very general terms how the process of producing health is related to the demand for health and the market for medical care. Actual statistical estimation of the parameters of the health production function requires addressing a number of empirical issues: the measurement of health, the choice of mortality as the health indicator for the analysis, the measurement of medical care use, the unit of analysis, choice of a mathematical form for the production function, data sources and file construction, and methods for dealing with several potential econometric problems (heteroskedasticity, specifications bias, and simultaneous equations bias). This chapter focuses on the first two of these issues. Though not necessarily less important, the other issues are discussed in Appendix A, Empirical Issues and Methods.

The Measurement of Health and Choice of Dependent Variables

It is generally agreed that health is a multidimensional concept which encompasses not only the absence of disease and disability but also the ability to carry out normal tasks and activities and to maintain an overall sense of well-being. It is also generally agreed that direct measurement of health is an elusive if not impossible task. In either case, there are essentially two approaches to measuring health empirically. One is to develop an index incorporating two or more of the components of a broad defini-

41

tion of health. The other is to designate a single item as an indicator or proxy for the health of a population. This section briefly discusses each of these approaches and presents a justification for the use of mortality as the dependent variable in subsequent analyses.

Construction of a health status index faces two major difficulties. One is simply defining a valid conceptual construct. In large part, this difficulty stems from the lack of a precise, unambiguous, and operational definition of health. Therefore, proposed health status indices must wrestle with which components of ill health ought to go into the index and how they should be weighted. Most likely, identification of valid indices will be the result of expert consensus rather than external or face validation.[1] The second difficulty impeding the development of a comprehensive health status index is the lack of requisite data, particularly at the level of small geographic areas.[2] Most proposed indices require data which can be collected only by means of household surveys or special questionnaires. While such data may be available at the national level through the Health Examination Survey, they are rarely available for small areas.[3]

Given the difficulties facing the development of health status indices, one should evaluate the potential utility for purposes of policy making of a much simpler indicator, namely mortality. Unlike most other indicators which might be combined to form a health status index, mortality is a unique and clearly defined event. There is no need to determine duration, intensity, or severity, all of which would have to be specified for various morbidity measures. The techniques for defining and reporting mortality data have been standardized to a point unmatched by methods for defining and reporting morbidity data. (This is not to say that there are no errors in mortality data, but only that the error rates are likely to be much lower than for morbidity measures.) Finally, and very importantly, mortality data are comparatively simple and widely understood by both policy makers and the general population. This last point could be critical to the acceptance of any health indicator or health status index as a legitimate tool in public policy making.

In support of these points, Whitmore argued that

> Appropriately classified, they (mortality data) provide a helpful profile of variations in health status throughout a population. The impact of a proposed health program, described in mortality terms, is readily assessed in a suitable cross-classification involving variables such as age, sex, race, geographical location, occupation, and the like. This is not to suggest that mortality is the only component of health. However, mortality is the most important and tractable of the components of health from the point of view of practical applica-

tion, and it must be understood before the theoretical foundations of other more refined approaches will be found.

A unique feature of the mortality component is that it arises in a uniform way at every decision-making level in the health field. The individual medical decision, the evaluation of a health program, and the determination of health care policy at the highest level all entail a consideration of mortality factors.[4]

Kohn makes a similar point with regard to evaluating health programs.

Traditionally and even at our present stage of knowledge, lower mortality has generally been regarded as an indication of better health. This is justifiable by and large; though mortality data do not tell the whole health story, declining mortality means a reduction in the final and most severe consequence of ill health. It is true that where we succeed today in prolonging the life of many patients without always curing their disease, we do not achieve health as such, but postponing mortality is no doubt an improvement in itself.

"Where there is life, there is hope": once we have extended life there is always the possibility, or hope, of a cure or of arresting the disease process. Similarly we can speak of improving health if we succeed, for instance, by rehabilitation procedures to change a disabling to a nondisabling or less disabling condition. Reduced mortality then may not necessarily mean health but is at least the first step towards better health.[5]

As will be discussed, there are a number of ways in which crude mortality data can be combined. This choice should be guided not only by the nature of the underlying disease processes or etiological factors but also by the proposed use and application of the measure. An index which may be superior along one dimension, say conceptual validity, is not necessarily superior for policy purposes. In particular, if *equally* good policy decisions can be made with less costly information, then the latter is clearly preferable for those purposes.

Aggregate mortality, of course, summarizes the results of many disease and social processes. It is quite likely, in fact, that cause-specific mortality rates differ in their sensitivity to both medical care use, personal characteristics, and area characteristics. Estimating the health production function for different types of mortality rates may provide useful information for the allocation of medical care resources among diseases. Therefore, in addition to investigating mortality rates from all causes combined, we shall also disaggregate the mortality data into deaths from external causes (accidents, homicides, suicides) and all natural causes, and further subdivide the latter into deaths from cancer (all sites), ischemic heart disease (acute and chronic), and all cardiovascular diseases.

A final word is in order regarding the quality of the mortality data. Probably the two major concerns about mortality statistics are their completeness and the accuracy of the recorded cause of death. Colby has conducted a thorough review of the literature regarding these issues.[6] With regard to the first, there is evidence that some deaths may be unreported in remote, geographically inaccessible areas. This is not likely to be a meaningful source of bias for this study because of the minimum population size of 250,000 for a county group.

The accuracy of the reported cause of death is of greater concern, however. Ambiguities in the face of multiple diseases, variations in the sophistication and extent of diagnostic techniques, and simple interphysician differences in custom may make geographic comparisons in cause-specific death rates hazardous. Several studies which attempted to verify the reported cause of death for individual causes found rates of agreement on the order of 70 to 80 percent.[7] Whether this rate is sufficiently high to validate the analysis of the cause-specific rates, assuming that their accuracy is about the same, cannot be assessed on a priori grounds. Grouping deaths by *major* cause of death categories should help reduce the potential error.

Three Approaches to the Measurement of Medical Care

The theoretical model developed in chapter 2 suggested that the medical care component of the health production function should be measured in terms of the quantities of the various medical care services used, for example, numbers of visits to physicians, days of hospitalization, and drug prescriptions. Ideally, these measures should be adjusted to account for variations in the quality and content of services: a visit to a specialist should probably be treated differently from a visit to a general practitioner, as should a day in a teaching hospital relative to a day in a nonteaching hospital. Unfortunately, data on the use of medical care are not generally available at either the county or county group level. Only two types of data are available at the county level: measures of the stocks of medical care providers—physicians, nurses, and hospital facilities—located in the county, and expenditures by Medicare for its enrolled population.

The medical care variables used in the empirical analysis must be constructed from these sources. Three approaches will be tested in the estimation of the adult cohorts' health production functions and two in the infant cohorts' functions. The remainder of this chapter and the next chapter consider only the adult cohorts. All results for infants are reported in chapter 6.

The first approach is based on stocks of resources in the county. These measures are of direct policy interest because most assessments of the adequacy of the local physician supply are derived from simple physician-to-population ratios. Therefore, medical care will be measured simply as the numbers of physicians, nurses, and hospital beds per 1,000 population in each county group. Total stocks will be adjusted to account for variations in the rates of nonpatient care activities, labor force participation, and excess capacity. Thus, the variables used in the analysis are based on the following subsets of the total stocks of medical care resources:

1. active, nonfederal patient care physicians (excluding interns);
2. active, registered and licensed practical nurses employed in hospital and nonhospital settings; and
3. occupied beds in all short-term, nonfederal, general hospitals.

Although this approach is the most straightforward, it has several apparent shortcomings. The health production functions will be estimated with data for age-sex-race-specific population cohorts, while the medical care variables are defined for the entire population. Cross-sectional variations in provider productivity partially offset variations in provider availability. As a result, the differences across areas in the per capita use of medical care services are likely to be overstated. Finally, measures based on these stocks of providers probably do not account very well for variations in the composition and quality of the services provided.

The second approach to measuring medical care is based on a method of allocating the stocks of providers among the age-sex-race cohorts. If one assumes that productivity in supplying physician visits and hospital days is constant across cohorts, it then follows that the share of the stock of resources available to a particular cohort is identical to the group's share of total physician visits or hospital days.

Information on medical care use (physician visits and hospital days) was obtained from the 1968 and 1970 Health Interview Surveys conducted by The National Center for Health Statistics. These data were stratified by census division, SMSA/non-SMSA residence, age, sex, and race using the same age-sex-race groupings applied to the mortality data. For each census division and place-of-residence combination, the ratios of physician visits and hospital days for each population cohort to all visits and hospital days were computed, that is,

$$VS_{icr} = V_{icr}/V_{cr} \tag{4.1}$$

where

VS_{icr} = physician visits *share* for the *ith* age-sex-race cohort in the *cth* census division and *rth* place of residence,

V_{icr} = physician visits by *ith* cohort in *cth* census division and *rth* place of residence, and

V_{cr} = total physician visits in *cth* census division and *rth* place of residence.

A similar set of weights was computed for hospital days, DS_{icr}.[8]

These weights were then applied to the total stock data for counties grouped by census division and SMSA status. VS_{icr} was applied to the physician and nonhospital nurse stock, while DS_{icr} was applied to the hospital nurse and occupied bed stocks. County data were then aggregated to the county group level, with each population cohort having the appropriate share of the total available stocks of physicians, nurses, and hospital beds assigned to it.

The other measurement problems mentioned can be dealt with only indirectly at best. Variations by size of place and region in visits per physician, average length of stay in hospitals, and the composition of services are well documented.[9] It is also suspected that the quality of care varies across areas, but defining and measuring quality are extremely difficult. In part, this is because quality has several dimensions: skill and accuracy in making diagnoses and applying treatments, personal and humane attention, more ancillary services per visit, the availability of the most sophisticated technologies, and the use of the most current diagnostic techniques. We shall attempt to control for these factors by the use of four proxy variables: the percentage of physicians who are general practitioners, the proportion of occupied hospital beds in hospitals with 11 or more facilities and services listed in the American Hospital Association's Annual Survey,[10] the presence of a medical school, and the number of foreign-graduated interns and residents per capita.

The third approach to measuring medical care is both the most parsimonious and probably the most defensible method on a priori grounds. Very simply, we shall assume that Medicare expenditures per Medicare enrollee are a constant proportion (across geographic areas) of medical care expenditures per capita in each population cohort. Under certain assumptions about the mathematical form of the health production function, it can be shown that the estimated coefficient of the medical care variable is invariant with respect to a scalar transformation. (See Appendix A for a proof of this proposition.) Thus, if the proportionality assumption can be justified, then the coefficient of the variable measuring Medicare expenditures per enrollee can be interpreted as an estimate of the coefficient of the age-sex-race-specific measure of per capita medical care expenditures.

Although only indirect evidence is available, it is consistent with the assumption stated. State data for 1970 were obtained for medical care expenditures per capita and Medicare expenditures per enrollee.[11] The former were limited to expenditures for physicians' services, hospital services, and prescription drugs.[12] Letting ME = Medicare expenditures per enrollee and MC = medical care expenditures per capita, the following two equations were estimated by ordinary least squares regressions:

$$ME = \beta \cdot MC \quad \text{and} \tag{4.2a}$$

$$ME = \alpha + \beta \cdot MC \tag{4.2b}$$

Using the sums of squared residuals from the two equations to compute an F-statistic, the null hypothesis that $\alpha = 0$ was not rejected.[13] The estimated value of β in equation (4.2a) is 2.476, which implies that Medicare expenditures per enrollee were approximately 2.5 times greater than medical care expenditures per capita in each state in 1970.[14]

Data on expenditures by age, sex, and race are much less readily available. However, examining data for two age groups (19 to 64, and 65 and older) for three years (1969-1971) and three services (physicians, hospitals, and drugs) suggests that the ratio of age-specific expenditures per capita to total expenditures per capita varies little over time and by service.[15] The biggest change in any of the ratios computed was 5.8 percent for hospital expenditures for the 65 and older population. Together, these findings support the assumption that Medicare expenditures per enrollee are constant proportion of age-sex-race-specific medical care expenditures per capita.

Several other factors make expenditures a more desirable measure of medical care use than either of the stocks-of-providers approaches. First, expenditures are a simple linear transformation of the theoretically desirable variables, quantities of services, that is, $MC = \sum_{i=1}^{n} P_i Q_i$, where the Q_i are quantities of individual services and the P_i are their prices. Stocks of providers are related to quantities through a much more complicated set of relationships, medical care production functions of the general form $Q_i = f_i(MD_i, N_i, B_i, Z_i)$, where MD_i = doctors, N_i = nurses, B_i = hospital beds, and Z_i = all other relevant factors.

Second, variations in expenditures are probably more closely related to variations in the quantity and quality of services used than are variations in the stocks of providers. Although there are cross-sectional variations in prices which are related to differences in the costs of providing care, these are small relative to the interarea variation in provider availability.[16] Furthermore price variations may reflect both quality and cost-of-living variations. Although one would like to adjust for the second component, there is no simple way of doing so with currently available data.

Third, Medicare expenditures per enrollee are reported for beneficiaries' place of residence (county and state). Thus, these data are much less likely to be subject to error because of border-crossing to obtain medical care and because of differences in providers' relevant trade areas. For example, many residents of suburban or rural counties may obtain their medical care from providers located in neighboring county groups. At the same time, differences in the specialty mix of physicians across county groups imply that the size of the relevant trade area may extend beyond a county group's boundaries.

Finally, Medicare expenditures per enrollee is the most parsimonious of the three proposed approaches for measuring medical care use. The other two methods require measures of the stocks of three medical care providers plus the use of one or more quality proxies. Even the theoretically desirable variables, quantities of different types of services use, require including several medical care variables in the production function. The fact that these multiple measures are likely to be highly correlated can lead to serious multicollinearity problems.

The apparent advantages of Medicare expenditures per enrollee as the measure of medical care use are clear. Nevertheless, the production functions will also be estimated using two measures of the stocks of providers per 1,000 people—the first set defined for the entire population and the second disaggregated to a cohort-specific level. These are of interest because of the common use of provider-to-population ratios in making public policy decisions about medical care resource allocation.

Empirical Tests of Alternative Medical Care Measures

This section reports the parameter estimates of the alternative measures of medical care use from the adult cohorts' health production functions.

As is discussed in more detail in Appendix A, it is reasonable to limit the evaluation of the alternative medical care measures to two possible mathematical forms of the production function, the Cobb-Douglas (CD), and the modified Cobb-Douglas (MDC) forms. The first constrains medical care's impact on mortality rates to always have the same sign, presumably negative. The second form allows medical care to have both negative and positive effects on the mortality rate. For example, increasing the use of medical care may continually reduce mortality rates up to some point. Further medical care consumption, however, may have no additional impact on mortality or, in some cases, might even lead to higher mortality rates because of iatrogenic factors. Based on the theory in chapter 2, it is also reasonable to explore whether medical care use and mortality rates are simultaneously determined, that is, although medical care use affects health levels, health levels also influence medical care use.

Consequently, the values of the medical care coefficients reported in tables 6 and 7 are for both the CD and MDC functional forms and are estimated by both single equation (OLS) and simultaneous equation (IV) methods. The complete equations include the final set of independent variables reported in chapter 5 and are estimated with data for pooled 10-year age cohorts within each sex-race combination. (See Appendix A for details.) The dependent variable in all of the equations is the natural logarithm of the mortality rate from all causes of death.

Two criteria, plausibility and statistical reliability, are used to evaluate the estimates. In general, one would expect the medical care variables to have negative coefficients in the CD form. In the MDC form, which includes both logarithmic and natural values of the medical care measures, the logarithmic value should have a negative coefficient and the natural value a positive coefficient. (This pattern of signs implies that increased medical care use reduces mortality rates by successively smaller decrements and eventually reaches a point of no impact on mortality.) Statistical reliability refers to the degree of confidence that can be attached to the inference that the estimated coefficient is not equal to zero. Although there are no firm guidelines, the 90 percent confidence level is usually treated as the minimally acceptable level of statistical reliability.

Table 6 reports the male cohorts' estimates for the two physician stock measures, physicians per 1,000 population in the county group (MDPOP) and physicians per 1,000 cohort members (MDCRT), and Medicare expenditures per enrollee (MDCREXP). Table 7 reports the same variables' coefficients for the female cohorts. Including measures of the stocks of nurses and hospital beds in the equations with the stock of physicians creates severe multicollinearity. This causes the estimates to become ex-

TABLE 6

COEFFICIENTS OF ALTERNATIVE MEDICAL CARE MEASURES[a,b]

Age Group and Variables	White Males				Black Males			
	Cobb-Douglas		Modified Cobb-Douglas		Cobb-Douglas		Modified Cobb-Douglas	
	OLS[c]	IV[d]	OLS	IV	OLS	IV	OLS	IV
45 to 64								
LMDPOP	.012	.002	.004	−.023	.067*	.084*	.104**	−.010
MDPOP			.006	.021			−.028	−.044
LMDCRT	.063*	.077*	.073	.051	.029*	.013	.063*	.066*
MDCRT			−.005	.012			−.012*	−.030*
LMDCREXP	−.098*	−.317*	−.085	−.460*	−.067	.043	.131	−.457
MDCREXP			NS	NS			−.001	.002
65+								
LMDPOP	−.006	.004	−.025	−.037	.009	.011	−.028	.047
MDPOP			.015	.030**			.029	.042
LMDCRT	.036*	.051*	.057*	.033	−.009	−.030*	−.039*	−.020
MDCRT			−.007	.005			−.007*	−.004
LMDCREXP	−.051*	−.123*	−.051*	−.457*	−.165*	−.166*	.084	−.675*
MDCREXP			NS	.001*			−.001	.002**

Key: MDPOP—Physicians per 1,000 population.
MDCRT—Physicians per 1,000 cohort members.
MDCREXP—Medicare expenditures per enrollee.
LMDPOP—Log MDPOP.
LMDCRT—Log MDCRT.
LMDCREXP—Log MDCREXP.

* Significant at 99 percent confidence level.
** Significant at 95 percent confidence level.
NS No significant digits.
a. Dependent variable is the log of the mortality rate for all causes of death.
b. See table 9 for a list of the other independent variables.
c. Ordinary least squares.
d. Instrumental variables.

TABLE 7

COEFFICIENTS OF ALTERNATIVE MEDICAL CARE MEASURES[a,b]

Age Group and Variables	White Females				Black Females			
	Cobb-Douglas		Modified Cobb-Douglas		Cobb-Douglas		Modified Cobb-Douglas	
	OLS[c]	IV[d]	OLS	IV	OLS	IV	OLS	IV
45 to 64								
LMDPOP	−.020	−.028†	.060*	.032	−.020	.006	−.011	−.014
MDPOP			−.006*	−.047*			−.007	.014
LMDCRT	−.007	.016	.095*	.048	−.048*	−.040*	−.015	.060*
MDCRT			−.038*	−.013			−.007**	−.032*
LMDCREXP	−.055**	−.126*	.372*	.726*	−.149*	−.108	.229	−.108
MDCREXP			−.001*	−.003*			−.001	NS
65+								
LMDPOP	−.028*	−.032*	−.008	−.041†	−.037	−.013	−.086	−.061
NDPOP			.023	.006			.039	.034
LMDCRT	−.010	−.018†	.052*	−.036	−.052*	−.046*	−.023	−.019
MDCRT			−.020	.006			−.008*	−.009
LMDCREXP	−.079*	−.141*	−.042	−.186	−.169*	−.183*	−.063	−.904*
MDCREXP			NS	NS			NS	.002**

Key: MDPOP—Physicians per 1,000 population.
 MDCRT—Physicians per 1,000 cohort members.
 MDCREXP—Medicare expenditures per enrollee.
 LMDPOP—Log MDPOP.
 LMDCRT—Log MDCRT.
 LMDCREXP—Log MDCREXP.

* Significant at 99 percent confidence level.
** Significant at 95 percent confidence level.
† Significant at 90 percent confidence level.
NS No significant digits.
a. Dependent variable is the log of the mortality rate for all causes of death.
b. See table 9 for a list of the other independent variables.
c. Ordinary least squares.
d. Instrumental variables.

tremely unreliable. (See Appendix A for the coefficient values for these specifications.)

As expected on theoretical grounds, an examination of the coefficients in these two tables strongly suggests that Medicare expenditures per enrollee is the best measure of medical care use for estimating health production functions. Seven of the eight coefficients in the Cobb-Douglas (CD) functional form have the predicted negative sign and are also statistically significant, generally at the 99 percent confidence level. Only one coefficient (black males, 45 to 64 years old, IV estimate) has a positive sign, but it is not statistically significant. In the modified Cobb-Douglas (MDC) form, the results are also highly consistent with prior expectations under IV estimation. Seven of eight pairs of coefficients have the correct signs and five are also statistically significant. The OLS estimates are much less plausible. Finally, the magnitude of the coefficients are very similar to the estimates of $-.065$ (OLS) and $-.116$ (IV) reported by Auster et al., who used state cross-section data for 1960 to estimate a health production function for whites.[17] Their health indicator was the age-sex-adjusted mortality rate for all causes of death, and their medical care measure was health expenditures per capita.

In contrast to these results, the coefficients of the physicians-per-1000-population (MDPOP) and physicians-per-1000-cohort-member (MDCRT) variables are both less plausible and less reliable. Five of eight coefficients have negative signs in the CD-OLS estimates for both measures. However, only two of the LMDCRT coefficients and one of the LMDPOP coefficients are also statistically significant. The best set of estimates for these two variables is the CD-IV combination for LMDCRT, which is both negative and statistically significant in four of the eight cases. No more than two coefficients satisfy these criteria for any of the other functional form and estimation method combinations.

Thus, both the theoretical arguments of the previous section and the empirical evidence presented in tables 6 and 7 support the use of Medicare expenditures per enrollee as the proxy for medical care use in the health production functions. The choices of a specific functional form and estimation method are complicated because no one combination of functional form and method is clearly superior to the other possibilities. As is detailed in Appendix A, however, the Cobb-Douglas form estimated by a simultaneous equation (IV) technique seems to provide the best mix of simplicity, plausibility, and statistical reliability.

5

HEALTH PRODUCTION FUNCTION ESTIMATES: ADULT COHORTS

This chapter presents the results of estimating health production functions for eight adult cohorts. The first section of the chapter lists the dependent and independent variables. This specification of the health production function consists of a subset of a larger, more comprehensive set of potential variables. (Those which were consistently statistically insignificant in preliminary estimations were deleted. See Appendix A.)

The second section reports the functions' parameter estimates. Mortality rates for all causes of death, external causes, all cancers, cardiovascular diseases, and ischemic heart disease are analyzed in addition to deaths from natural causes. The primary focus of this section is the impact of medical care on mortality, although the effects of other factors are also discussed.

Empirical Specifications

1. THE MORTALITY RATES

As discussed in the previous chapter, various mortality rates are used as health indicators in the health production function specifications. The most inclusive indicator is the mortality rate from all causes of death. One obvious problem with this particular indicator is that it includes some causes of death which may not be very susceptible to medical treatment. For example, many deaths from external causes such as homicide, suicide, and automobile accidents, may occur before any medical treatments

53

can be administered and may have little relationship to prior medical care use. Among natural causes of death, some disease groups, particularly cancers, are thought to be "incurable," that is, there is very little case-specific evidence that medical treatment can alter the course of the disease.

These observations suggest that the impact of medical care on mortality rates is likely to vary across cause-of-death groups. In order to investigate this hypothesis, mortality rates from all causes are first subdivided into rates from all natural causes and all external causes of deaths. In addition, three specific subsets of natural causes are also analyzed: the mortality rates from all cancers, cardiovascular diseases, and ischemic heart diseases. Between 1960 and 1970, the age-adjusted mortality rates for the last two groups decreased by about 16 and 12 percent, respectively.[1] In contrast to these declines, the age-adjusted mortality rates for cancers and accidents each increased by about 4 percent.[2] Thus, if medical care does have an effect on mortality rates, it is much more likely to be identifiable for the cardiovascular and ischemic heart disease causes of death. In addition, a comparison of medical care's impact across the different causes of death provides an indication of the validity of Medicare expenditures per enrollee as a measure of medical care expenditures per cohort member. If it is a good proxy, then its coefficients should be largest in the cardiovascular and ischemic heart disease mortality rate equations, smallest in the external causes and cancer mortality rate equations, and larger in the all natural causes equation than in the all causes equation.

Table 8 reports the mean values of the alternative mortality rates for each of the 8 adult cohorts in the analysis. As is well known, mortality rates are lower for females than for males, and for whites than for blacks in each age grouping. Deaths from external causes account for a higher proportion of deaths among the younger cohorts and the male cohorts. Except for middle-aged females, cardiovascular diseases are responsible for between 50 and 60 percent of deaths.

2. MEDICAL CARE

As discussed in the previous chapter and Appendix A, medical care use is approximated by Medicare expenditures per enrollee. This measure is assumed to be proportional to actual per capita medical care expenditures in each cohort. Since health and medical care use appear to be simultaneously determined, an instrumental variable approach is used to construct the medical care variables actually included in the regression analysis. For white cohorts, the instrumental variable is the predicted value of the

TABLE 8

MEAN MORTALITY RATES BY CAUSE OF DEATH,
ADULT COHORTS: DEATHS PER 1,000 PEOPLE[a]

CAUSE OF DEATH	ICDA CODES	WHITE MALES, 45-64	BLACK MALES, 45-64	WHITE MALES, 65+	BLACK MALES, 65+	WHITE FEMALES, 45-64	BLACK FEMALES, 45-64	WHITE FEMALES, 65+	BLACK FEMALES, 65+
All causes		13.86	22.82	75.81	72.30	6.57	13.88	46.09	51.30
External causes	800-999	1.29	2.41	2.36	2.23	0.46	0.58	1.18	0.99
Natural causes	000-796	12.42	20.05	73.46	69.86	6.07	13.19	44.87	50.21
All cancers	140-209	2.82	4.18	12.39	12.18	2.31	2.95	6.98	6.45
Ischemic heart disease	410-413	5.43	6.01	31.71	24.30	1.30	3.29	18.31	18.26
Cardiovascular disease	390-448	6.87	9.92	46.72	41.78	2.21	6.34	29.50	33.33

a. Unweighted means of county groups.

logarithm of Medicare expenditures per enrollee. For black cohorts, the actual value of the logarithm of Medicare expenditures per enrollee is assumed to be an appropriate instrumental variable, since its value is determined primarily by whites' medical care consumption patterns.

Variations in the quality and accessibility of medical care are assumed to be related to a crude but simple indicator, the difference between cohort-specific actual and predicted death rates from influenza and pneumonia (EXFLU). The predicted rate is based on each cohort's socio-demographic and health stock characteristics, and the area characteristics of the county group. It is assumed that the greater the number of actual flu and pneumonia deaths in excess of predicted rates, the lower the quality and/or accessibility of the medical care used by that cohort.

3. INITIAL HEALTH STATUS

As noted in chapter 2, variations across cohorts in initial health status can affect both the efficiency of health production and the demands for health and medical care. Therefore, it is important to control for these variations in order to obtain unbiased estimates of the relationship between medical care use and mortality.[3] Since direct measures of health status are not available, two groups of proxy variables will be used. One measures behavior which might be indicative of differences in health status. The other group consists of possible underlying sources of variations in health status.

Included in the first group are the decisions to participate in the labor force and to move from place to place. These are used as measures of differences in health status because people in poor health are less likely to be in the labor force and less likely to make an interstate move than people in good health. Separate measures of labor force participation are used for men and women: the proportion of men not in the labor force in 1970 who reported that they last worked in 1968 or later (WORK68), and the proportion of women not in the labor force (NILF). The migration rate is defined as the proportion of cohort members who resided in a different state five years earlier (MIGR). Finally, childbearing experience is also used as an indicator of women's health, on the grounds that women in poor health are likely to have fewer children than women in good health. This variable is defined as the average number of children ever born (KIDS).

The second group of health status proxies consists of possible sources of variations in health status. These include age, sex, race, and nativity. The first three factors are controlled for primarily through the stratification of the population into separate age-sex-race-specific cohorts. However, since the health production functions will be estimated for pairs of cohorts pooled by age intervals, age will also be measured by the average age (AVA) of the pooled cohorts. Nativity will be measured by the proportion of cohort members born in the United States (USB). Finally, two additional indicators of health status are the proportion of armed forces veterans (VET) and the proportion of cohort members reporting a work-limiting or work-preventing disability (DISABL). The former, which is defined only for males, may measure service-related injuries or ill health. The latter is the only direct measure of health from the 1970 Census. Unfortunately, it was asked only of people under the age of 65.

4. BEHAVIOR/LIFE-STYLE

Direct measures of key aspects of health behavior, such as diet, smoking, alcohol consumption, exercise, and rest are not available for small geographic areas. An indirect proxy for variations in alcohol consumption is constructed from an estimate of the expected number of deaths from cirrhosis of the liver and alcohol consumption by cohort and area.[4] The difference between the actual and expected death rates (EXALCIR) is then interpreted as an index of the effects of alcohol consumption. A second behavioral variable measures crude differences in cigarette consumption. It is defined as the number of cigarettes sold per capita (CIGS) in each state in 1970. Unfortunately, no data are available by age, sex, and race, nor is it possible to distinguish sales from consumption. It is important, therefore, to interpret both of these variables as indicators of differences in behavior rather than as direct measures of alcohol or cigarette consumption. The key assumption is that areas with relatively large values of EXALCIR and CIGS are also likely to have relatively high alcohol and cigarette consumption. Thus, both should have positive signs in the health production functions.

Four variables are included as general measures of differences in life-style. These are education, defined as the average highest grade attended (AHG) by the cohort, average total income of cohort members' families (TFI), the proportion of the cohort which is currently married (MAR), and, for the male cohorts, the proportion employed in agriculture (AGR). These factors have frequently been found to be significantly related to variations in mortality rates. All are expected to have negative associations with mortality rates.

Education is hypothesized to affect health production efficiency. Holding other factors, especially medical care use, constant, higher education levels should be associated with lower mortality rates. Higher family incomes imply both a greater ability to purchase goods and services, such as shelter, food, clothing, and recreation, which have positive effects on health, and possibly a greater demand for health. Thus, shifts in both the health production function and the health demand function should lead to a negative association with mortality rates.

The marital status variable measures several factors. First, it is assumed to be related to the caring and support functions provided by spouses and possibly to differences in attitudes toward risky behavior. Second, marriage may also be an indirect indicator of underlying health status, since people in poor health are probably less likely to marry than people in good health. Third, widowhood and divorce, particularly among older people, may be significant sources of emotional stress, which in turn leads to poorer health. Finally, agricultural employment may reflect lower health risks associated both with farming and with rural residence.

5. ENVIRONMENT

Variables measuring environmental characteristics focus on water quality, air quality, climate, and occupational hazards. Because these factors are unlikely to be strongly associated with the consumption of medical care, the choice of specific measures is guided primarily by data availability. Water quality will be measured by two variables: the percentage of households which obtain water from public systems (PWS) and the percentage of households with public sewer connections (PSC). Climate is measured by three variables: mean January temperature (MJT), mean annual precipitation (RAIN), and mean annual percentage sunshine (SUN). Air quality is approximated by an index of suspended particles in the air (PARTS). Finally, exposure to occupational hazards is measured by the proportion of cohort members in "hazardous industries"—mining, construction, chemical, rubber, paper, and metal smelting industries (HIND). This variable is defined only for male cohorts. One would expect a high index of suspended particles and a high proportion of workers in hazardous industries to be positively associated with mortality rates. However, there are no prior expectations about the signs of the other variables.

Data for three of the environmental variables, RAIN, SUN, and PARTS, are available only for a limited number of measuring stations. Rather than restrict the entire analysis to only those areas, the impact of environmental factors is explored in two stages. The first uses only those environmental measures which are available for all of the county groups. In a subsequent section, the effects of the additional environmental variables are examined, albeit for a reduced number of observations.

The means and standard deviations of the final set of independent variables are presented in table 9. The mean of the log of Medicare expenditures per enrollee (LMDCREXP) is approximately the same across cohorts since it is not constructed as an age-sex-race-specific variable. Two other variables, cigarettes sold per capita per year (CIGS) and mean January temperature (MJT) are also defined for the county group rather than for each cohort.[5] The latter is consistently larger for blacks than for whites, reflecting the fact that there are few blacks in many of the north central and mountain states. The other variables generally follow expected patterns of male-female and black-white differences in demographic characteristics.

Health Production Function Estimates

1. DEATHS FROM ALL CAUSES

Tables 10 and 11 present the parameters of the health production functions for males and females, respectively. The dependent variable is the natural log of the mortality rate for deaths from all causes. Overall, the equations explain extremely high proportions of the geographic variation in mortality rates: between 95 and 98 percent of the variation in whites'

TABLE 9

MEANS AND STANDARD DEVIATIONS OF FINAL INDEPENDENT VARIABLES, ADULT COHORTS

(STANDARD DEVIATION IN PARENTHESES)

	WHITE MALES, 45–64	BLACK MALES, 45–64	WHITE MALES, 65+	BLACK MALES, 65+
LMDCREXP[a]	5.68 (0.17)	5.69 (0.24)	5.68 (0.17)	5.65 (0.23)
AVA	54.28 (4.92)	54.21 (4.99)	74.64 (5.65)	73.52 (5.93)
EXFLU[c]	0.0020(0.16)	0.0080(0.43)	0.0017(0.16)	0.0003(0.28)
USB (%)	95.59 (5.03)	98.82 (3.07)	86.93 (12.50)	98.51 (4.45)
WORK68 (%)	10.89 (4.43)	13.25 (7.11)	17.20 (7.11)	15.75 (9.90)
VET (%)	25.78 (11.39)	20.55 (12.16)	13.16 (3.72)	10.28 (6.57)
MIGR (%)	2.97 (2.61)	1.79 (3.08)	2.18 (2.67)	1.20 (2.58)
DISABL (%)[b]	10.13 (3.37)	12.60 (4.62)	NA	NA
NILF (%)	NA	NA	NA	NA
KIDS	NA	NA	NA	NA
CIGS (00's)	23.78 (3.72)	23.96 (3.78)	23.78 (3.72)	23.72 (4.00)
EXALCIR[c]	0.0001(0.09)	0.0026(0.38)	−0.0057(0.74)	−0.248 (0.91)
AHG	12.61 (1.11)	9.72 (1.66)	10.48 (1.14)	7.21 (1.50)
TFI ($00's)	117.91 (26.33)	72.77 (23.22)	65.69 (19.61)	39.37 (13.78)
MAR (%)	88.09 (3.44)	73.57 (8.75)	72.41 (9.92)	59.81 (13.18)
AGR (%)	8.40 (8.73)	8.76 (10.67)	9.90 (8.70)	11.57 (11.97)
MJT	34.94 (11.51)	40.08 (10.73)	34.94 (11.51)	43.03 (9.93)
PWS (%)	36.25 (8.98)	40.00 (13.63)	36.43 (9.67)	36.95 (14.33)
HIND (%)	23.72 (9.12)	23.65 (12.06)	12.22 (7.39)	10.95 (10.08)

TABLE 9 (cont'd)

	White Females, 45–64	Black Females, 45–64	White Females, 65+	Black Females, 65+
LMDCREXP[a]	5.68　(0.17)	5.68　(0.23)	5.68　(0.17)	5.64　(0.23)
AVA	54.33　(4.97)	54.20　(5.08)	74.80　(5.67)	74.07　(6.23)
EXFLU[c]	0.0006(0.08)	0.0072(0.23)	−0.0002(0.07)	0.0014(0.74)
USB (%)	95.33　(5.10)	98.94　(3.09)	89.18 (10.79)	98.94　(3.78)
WORK68 (%)	NA	NA	NA	NA
VET (%)	NA	NA	NA	NA
MIGR (%)	2.89　(2.52)	1.84　(2.75)	2.31　(2.45)	1.23　(2.39)
DISABL (%)[b]	8.41　(2.66)	13.25　(3.95)	NA	NA
NILF (%)	36.17　(7.98)	27.03 (11.14)	73.76 (12.05)	66.12 (15.87)
KIDS	2.51　(0.40)	3.07　(0.83)	2.81　(0.64)	3.13　(0.91)
CIGS (00's)	23.78　(3.72)	23.85　(3.71)	23.78　(3.72)	23.58　(3.92)
EXALCIR[c]	0.0003(0.05)	−0.0043(0.22)	−0.0057(0.50)	0.0054(0.61)
AHG	12.72　(0.88)	10.46　(1.31)	10.98　(1.01)	8.11　(1.41)
TFI ($00's)	103.76 (26.29)	62.18 (23.58)	58.63 (17.19)	37.20 (16.07)
MAR (%)	75.72　(7.62)	56.55 (10.62)	35.27 (13.58)	27.22 (12.35)
AGR (%)	NA	NA	NA	NA
MJT	34.94 (11.51)	40.32 (10.64)	34.94 (11.51)	41.83 (10.01)
PWS (%)	37.43　(8.39)	40.80 (11.81)	39.16　(7.99)	40.17 (14.27)
HIND (%)	NA	NA	NA	NA

a. Natural log, predicted value for white cohorts.
b. Instrumental variable.
c. Computed as the difference between actual and predicted mortality rates.
NA Not applicable.
Key: LMDCREXP—Log Medicare expenditures per enrollee.
　　　AVA—Average age in years.
　　　EXFLU—Excess deaths from flu and pneumonia.
　　　USB—Percentage U.S. born.
　　　WORK68—Percentage last worked between 1968 and 1970.
　　　VET—Percentage veterans.
　　　MIGR—Percentage resided in a different state in 1965.
　　　DISABL—Percentage reporting an activity-limiting disability.
　　　NILF—Percentage not in labor force.
　　　KIDS—Average number of children ever born.
　　　CIGS—Cigarettes sold per capita (in state).
　　　EXALCIR—Excess deaths from alcoholism and cirrhosis.
　　　AHG—Average highest grade completed.
　　　TFI—Total income per family.
　　　MAR—Percentage married.
　　　AGR—Percentage in agriculture.
　　　MJT—Mean January temperature.
　　　PWS—Percentage with water from public systems.
　　　HIND—Percentage employed in hazardous industries.

TABLE 10

REGRESSION COEFFICIENTS: DEATHS FROM ALL CAUSES
(ADULT MALE COHORTS)

VARIABLES	WHITE MALES, 45–64	BLACK MALES, 45–64	WHITE MALES, 65+	BLACK MALES, 65+
LMDCREXP[a]	−.3242*	−.0772[†]	−.1233*	−.1632*
EXFLU	.1607*	.1004*	.0786*	.0019
AVA	.0850*	.0617*	.0741*	.0045*
USB	NS	−.0009	.0005	.0006
WORK68	−.0003	.0008	−.0019**	−.0016**
VET	.0017	−.0008	.0012	−.0019[†]
MIGR	−.0058*	−.0021	−.0093*	.0007
DISABL[a]	.0105*	−.0058**	NA	NA
AHG	−.0205*	−.0133[†]	−.0122*	−.0083
TFI	−.0006**	−.0016*	NS	−.0007
MAR	−.0146*	−.0017**	−.0021*	−.0004
AGR	−.0055*	−.0020**	−.0038*	−.0006
CIGS	.0055*	.0086*	.0027*	.0006*
EXALCIR	.1891*	.1698*	.0122**	.0336*
MJT	.0030*	.0034*	−.0008*	−.0009
PWS	.0024*	−.0003**	.0020*	.0019*
HIND	−.0007	.0021*	.0005	.0015[†]
R^2 (adj)	0.97	0.84	0.97	0.83
F	1321.45	128.31	1705.13	90.26
N	796	428	796	294

*Significant at 99 percent confidence level.
**Significant at 95 percent confidence level.
[†]Significant at 90 percent confidence level.
a. Instrumental variable.
NS Less than .0001.
NA Not applicable.
Key: LMDCREXP—Log Medicare expenditures per enrollee.
    EXFLU—Excess deaths from flu and pneumonia.
    AVA—Average age in years.
    USB—Percentage U.S. born.
    WORK68—Percentage last worked between 1968 and 1970.
    VET—Percentage veterans.
    MIGR—Percentage resided in a different state in 1965.
    DISABL—Percentage reporting an activity-limiting disability.
    AHG—Average highest grade completed.
    TFI—Total income per family.
    MAR—Percentage married.
    AGR—Percentage employed in agriculture.
    CIGS—Cigarettes sold per capita (in state).
    EXALCIR—Excess deaths from alcoholism and cirrhosis.
    MJT—Mean January temperature.
    PWS—Percentage with water from public systems.
    HIND—Percentage employed in hazardous industries.

TABLE 11

REGRESSION COEFFICIENTS: DEATHS FROM ALL CAUSES
(ADULT FEMALE COHORTS)

VARIABLES	WHITE FEMALES, 45–64	BLACK FEMALES, 45–64	WHITE FEMALES, 65+	BLACK FEMALES, 65+
LMDCREXP[a]	−.1254**	−.1543*	−.1414*	−.1728*
EXFLU	.3719*	.1571*	.1224*	.0049
AVA	.0586*	.0546*	.0915*	.0529*
USB	−.0072*	.0069**	−.0017*	.0021
MIGR	−.0031†	−.0043	−.0057*	−.0036
DISABL[a]	.0081	−.0068**	NA	NA
NILF	.0041*	.0017**	.0022*	.0003
KIDS	−.0531*	−.0459*	−.0348*	−.0365*
AHG	.0165**	−.0381*	−.0023*	−.0131
TFI	−.0003	.0003	−.0003	−.0003
MAR	−.0095*	−.0042*	−.0077*	−.0011
CIGS	.0045*	.0043**	.0023*	.0020
EXALCIR	.3870*	.1974*	.0133**	.0245†
MJT	−.0008†	.0056*	−.0024*	−.0006
PWS	.0013**	−.0004	−.0003	.0005
R^2 (adj)	0.95	0.83	0.98	0.84
F	1025.88	132.36	3571.18	112.53
N	796	412	796	302

*Significant at 99 percent confidence level.
**Significant at 95 percent confidence level.
†Significant at 90 percent confidence level.
a. Instrumental variable.
NA Not applicable.

Key: LMDCREXP—Log Medicare expenditures per enrollee.
       EXFLU—Excess deaths from flu and pneumonia.
       AVA—Average age in years.
       USB—Percentage U.S. born.
       MIGR—Percentage resided in a different state in 1965.
       DISABL—Percentage reporting an activity-limiting disability.
       NILF—Percentage not in labor force.
       KIDS—Average number of children ever born.
       AHG—Average highest grade completed.
       TFI—Total income per family.
       MAR—Percentage married.
       CIGS—Cigarettes sold per capita (in state).
       EXALCIR—Excess deaths from alcoholism and cirrhosis.
       MJT—Mean January temperature.
       PWS—Percentage with water from public systems.

rates, and 83 or 84 percent of the variation for blacks. About half of this explanatory power, however, is due to the variable measuring the average age (AVA) of the cohort. Since each 20-year cohort was constructed by pooling two 10-year cohorts, AVA is bimodal with peaks at approximately the midpoints of each 10-year age span. As such, it is essentially equivalent to a dichotomous variable which distinguishes the older from the younger age group within each cohort. (AVA was not statistically significant in equations estimated with data for 10-year age groups.)

Turning to the parameter estimates themselves, the coefficients of the log of Medicare expenditures per enrollee (LMDCREXP) strongly suggest that medical care use is a significant factor in explaining geographic variations in mortality rates. All coefficients are statistically significant at the 95 percent confidence level or higher. Except for middle-aged males, the magnitudes of the coefficients are remarkably similar across cohorts, ranging from $-.1233$ for white males 65 and older, to $-.1728$ for black females 65 and older. (Because of the functional form used, these coefficients are equivalent to elasticities, the percentage change in the mortality rate for a 1 percent change in medical care spending per capita.) The coefficient for white males 45 to 64, $-.3242$, is about twice as large as the coefficients for the other cohorts, while that for black males 45 to 64, $-.0772$, is about half as large. There is no readily apparent reason for the divergence of these two coefficients from the estimates for the other cohorts. On average, these parameters suggest that a 10 percent increase in medical care expenditures per capita will reduce adult mortality rates by about 1.5 percent.

The second medical care variable is EXFLU, the difference between the actual and expected mortality rates from influenza and pneumonia. It is included in the model as a proxy for the quality of medical care. As expected, all coefficients are positive and, except for the elderly black cohorts, also statistically significant at the 99 percent level of confidence. Since this is not a direct measure of medical care quality, however, it is not possible to draw any inferences about specific aspects of the medical care system.

Measures of health status are generally statistically significant and generally enter the equations with the expected signs. This is particularly true for the white cohorts. As noted, average age (AVA) is positive and statistically significant in each cohort. The average number of children ever born (KIDS) has the hypothesized negative coefficient and is statistically significant at the 99 percent confidence level in all four female cohorts, with somewhat larger effects in the equations for younger women. The percentage reporting an activity-limiting disability (DISABL), which was available only for the under age 65 cohorts, is positive and significant for both white cohorts but negative and significant for the black cohorts. Similarly, the percentage of the cohort which resided in a different state five years earlier (MIGR), has a negative sign and is statistically significant for all white cohorts but is significant only for one black cohort. (A high migration rate is assumed to be correlated with both good health and economic status.)

Two labor force participation variables are also assumed to be related to health and economic status. For males, the percentage not in the labor force who last worked in 1968, 1969, or 1970 (WORK68) is hypothesized to have a negative coefficient, that is, the more recent the departure from the labor force, the higher health status. For females, percentage not in the labor force (NILF) was expected to have a positive impact, although this might be confounded by a positive correlation between NILF and economic status. The variable for males has the expected negative coefficient in three of the four cohorts and is also statistically significant for the elderly cohorts. For females, NILF has a positive and significant coefficient for three of the cohorts. This suggests that the impact of health status on women's labor force participation may outweigh the effects of economic status. Finally, the last two health status proxies are the percentage U.S. born (USB) and the percentage of males who are veterans (VET). There were no prior expectations about their signs, and the results for these two variables do not suggest any clearcut patterns.

The variables measuring lifestyle or behavioral factors are also generally consistent with hypotheses about their effects on mortality rates. Of particular interest are the education and income variables, which have been the primary focus of several earlier studies. Education (AHG) has a negative coefficient in all but one equation (white females, 45 to 64) and is statistically significant for all cohorts except elderly blacks. Total family income (TFI) also has a negative coefficient in all but one cohort but is statistically significant only for younger males. These findings must be qualified, however, by the inevitable problem of a high degree of multicollinearity between income and education. (See chapter 7 for a more detailed analysis of the relationship between income and mortality.) Being married (MAR) and employment in the agriculture sector (AGR, males only) are also consistently associated with lower mortality rates.

Finally, two crude proxies for personal habits are cigarettes sold per capita (CIGS) and the difference between actual and expected mortality rates from alcoholism and cirrhosis of the liver (EXALCIR). The former is hypothesized to be a proxy for smoking and the latter for alcohol consumption. Both are predicted to have positive effects on mortality rates.

The coefficients of these variables strongly support these predictions. All have positive signs and all but one (for each variable) are statistically significant at the 90 percent confidence level or better.

It is also interesting to note that the coefficients for the younger cohorts are consistently larger in magnitude than those for the older cohorts. This may reflect the fact that the impacts of smoking and alcohol consumption are greater relative to other causes of death among nonelderly persons. In 1971, deaths from causes typically associated with smoking and alcohol consumption—cirrhosis of the liver, alcoholism, bronchitis, asthma, emphysema, and neoplasms of the respiratory system—accounted for 13.2 percent of deaths among 45 to 64 year olds but only 4.6 percent of deaths among those 65 and older.[6]

No estimate of the quantitative importance of alcohol consumption can be drawn from EXALCIR because it is not a direct measure of consumption levels. The coefficients of CIGS, on the other hand, suggest that to the extent that cigarette consumption is related to cigarette sales, a decrease in sales of 11.5 percent, from 2.3 to 2.0 packages sold per person per week, would reduce mortality rates by about 1.3 percent for females, 45 to 64, by 1.6 percent for white males, 45 to 64, and by 2.6 percent for black males, 45 to 64.[7] Presumably, the impact on smokers' mortality rates would be larger. Although these results are based on admittedly crude data, they are consistent with large volumes of other research on these issues.

The last three variables in the model are limited measures of environmental characteristics: mean January temperature (MJT), the percentage of cohort members with water from public systems (PWS), and, for males, the percentage employed in allegedly hazardous industries (HIND). No predictions were made about the first two, while the third was hypothesized to have a positive relationship with the mortality rate. This prediction is borne out to a limited extent. HIND is positive and statistically significant in both equations for black males but is not significant for white males. The results for MJT and PWS are also not clearcut. MJT's coefficients are negative for the elderly cohorts and positive for the younger cohorts, with six of the eight attaining statistical significance. However an examination of simple correlation coefficients shows that MJT is positively correlated with the migration rate (MIGR) for whites and negatively correlated with income (TFI) and education (AHG) for blacks. Thus, it appears that this variable may simply reflect regional differences in the distributions of the factors with which it is highly correlated. Similarly, PWS, which is positive and statistically significant in four equations is relatively highly correlated with factors usually associated with urban-rural population differences. As such, the positive coefficients may reflect higher mortality rates in urban areas rather than characteristics of the water consumed. Based on these results and on those reported for other environmental factors, it appears that no conclusions can be drawn in this study about the relationship between the environment and mortality rates without better data which directly measure relevant environmental characteristics.

2. MEDICAL CARE AND CAUSE-SPECIFIC MORTALITY RATES

The analysis of cause-specific mortality rates is motivated by two questions. First, does medical care have a differential impact on mortalities from different causes? Second, if it does, are there any implications for the allocation of medical care resources among disease groups? Since the measure of medical care use is Medicare expenditures per enrollee rather than cohort- and disease-specific expenditures, this phase of the analysis must be treated as exploratory.

Table 12 reports the coefficients of Medicare expenditures per enrollee for each of the mortality rates in the study.[8] Several patterns emerge from these results. First, deaths from external causes and all cancers appear to be less closely related to medical care use than deaths from ischemic and cardiovascular causes. However, since deaths from external causes are a relatively small proportion of all deaths, the coefficients in the deaths from natural causes equations are very similar to those for deaths from all causes.

Second, both cardiovascular and ischemic heart disease (which is responsible for about two-thirds of cardiovascular deaths) appear responsive to medical care use. For each of the white cohorts, the coefficient in the ischemic heart disease equation is larger in magnitude (by as much as 50 percent) than the coefficient in the cardiovascular disease equations; the reverse is true for the black cohorts. Furthermore, with one exception, the coefficients are larger for whites than for blacks. Coefficients are also larger for middle-aged whites than for elderly whites. The same pattern holds for black females, though not for black males. Finally, male-female differences in each age group appear smaller on average than black-white differences.

A third inference which emerges from table 12 is that within each cause category, mortality rates for middle-aged white males appear to be more sensitive to the use of medical care than those for any other cohort. This is true even in the equations for deaths from cancers and external causes, in which the medical care coefficients are not statistically significant and of the hypothesized sign for other cohorts. Middle-aged black males, on the

TABLE 12

ELASTICITY OF MORTALITY WITH RESPECT TO MEDICAL CARE BY CAUSE OF DEATH

(ADULT COHORTS)

CAUSE OF DEATH	WHITE MALES, 45–64	BLACK MALES, 45–64	WHITE MALES, 65+	BLACK MALES, 65+	WHITE FEMALES, 45–64	BLACK FEMALES, 45–64	WHITE FEMALES, 65+	BLACK FEMALES, 65+
All causes	−.3242*	−.0772†	−.1233*	−.1632*	−.1254*	−.1543*	−.1414*	−.1928*
External causes	−.2601**	−.0089	.1093	−.1704	.2432**	−.0027	.2402**	−.1967
Natural causes	−.3121*	−.0809†	−.1296*	−.1609*	−.1446*	−.1685*	−.1508*	−.1698*
Cancer	−.2033*	.1014	−.0342	.1515**	.0647	−.0410	.0751†	.0617
Ischemic heart disease	−.4767*	−.0724	−.3426*	−.1852*	−.5464*	−.2435**	−.4789*	−.0807
Cardiovascular disease	−.4167*	−.1458**	−.2489*	−.3012*	−.3761*	−.2416*	−.3085*	−.2152*

*Significant at 99 percent confidence level.
**Significant at 95 percent confidence level.
†Significant at 90 percent confidence level.

other hand, generally have the smallest medical care coefficients of all of the adult cohorts. These results for cause-specific mortality rates parallel those based on deaths from all causes. As noted, there is no ready explanation from the data in this study as to why the coefficients for these two cohorts should diverge from those for the other age-sex-race groups.

The impacts of other variables on cause-specific mortality rates generally parallel those reported in the analysis of deaths from all causes.[9] The coefficients of the variable measuring cigarette sales per capita (CIGS) are of particular interest, however, for two reasons. First, the relationship between smoking and health has been a subject of major controversy for more than 25 years. Second, the pattern of coefficient signs, magnitudes, and statistical significance may aid in assessing the validity of CIGS as a proxy for cigarette consumption.

Table 13 presents the coefficients (and elasticities) of CIGS by cohort and cause of death. Overall, the results seem consistent with the arguments advanced by the proponents of a link between cigarette smoking and health. First, only one coefficient is statistically significant in the equations for deaths from external causes. Second, all coefficients are positive, statistically significant (except one), and generally largest in magnitude in the equations for cardiovascular and ischemic heart disease. Third, cancer death rates are significantly and positively related to CIGS for males, but not for females. (Note that these data are for adults over the age of 44 in 1970 and thus reflect the much higher incidence of smoking among adult males than among adult females at that time.)[10] Finally, the elasticity estimates suggest that small reductions in cigarette sales per capita could result in significant reductions in mortality rates. In general, then, the consistency of these results with other commonly reported findings reinforces the interpretation of CIGS as a valid measure of cigarette consumption.

3. ENVIRONMENTAL FACTORS AND DEATHS FROM NATURAL CAUSES

One of the four general factors hypothesized to influence mortality rates is the environment. The problems of pollution and environmental health hazards are now major political and social issues. However, analysis of their effects on mortality rates is hampered by the lack of systematic identification and uniform measurement of relevant environmental characteristics. This is particularly true of data collected in 1970, when widespread concern about the environment was just beginning. As a result, this phase of the study must be limited to the particular measures available at the time. Furthermore, even these limited measures exist for only about one-third of the country groups.

TABLE 13

COEFFICIENTS OF CIGS BY CAUSE OF DEATH AND COHORT
(ELASTICITIES IN PARENTHESES)

CAUSE OF DEATH	WHITE MALES, 45–64	BLACK MALES, 45–64	WHITE MALES, 65+	BLACK MALES, 65+	WHITE FEMALES, 45–64	BLACK FEMALES, 45–64	WHITE FEMALES, 65+	BLACK FEMALES, 65+
External causes	.0027 (.063)	.0134* (.315)	.002 (.047)	.0098 (.230)	.0017 (.040)	−.0059 (−.139)	−.0002 (−.005)	.0089 (.209)
All natural causes	.0059* (.139)	.0077* (.181)	.0027* (.053)	.0057 (.134)	.0047* (.110)	.0048** (.113)	.0024* (.056)	.0019 (.045)
Cancers	.0064* (.150)	.0085** (.200)	.0021 (.049)	.0025 (.058)	.0013 (.031)	−.0014 (−.033)	−.0006 (−.014)	−.0021 (−.049)
Ischemic heart disease	.0079* (.186)	.011* (.259)	.0059* (.139)	.0163* (.383)	.0099* (.233)	.0142* (.334)	.0054* (.127)	.0119* (.280)
Cardiovascular disease	.0088* (.209)	.0062* (.146)	.0048* (.113)	.0094* (.221)	.0066* (.155)	.0068† (.160)	.0086 (.202)	.0049 (.115)

*Significant at 99 percent confidence level.
**Significant at 95 percent confidence level.
†Significant at 90 percent confidence level.

Table 14 reports the coefficients of seven environmental factors included in the model. These variables are hypothesized to represent four different elements of the environment: exposure to industrial pollutants (HIND—the proportion of cohort (males only) workers employed in hazardous industries); water system characteristics (PWS—the proportion of the cohort with water from public systems, and PSC—the proportion with public sewer connections); climatic conditions (SUN—mean annual percentage sunshine, RAIN—mean annual precipitation, and MJT—mean January temperature); and air quality (PARTS—90th percentile of suspended particulates measured in micrograms per cubic meter). The first three variables are constructed from data for cohort members, while the last four are based upon data for the entire county or county group.

Taken together, the set of seven variables generally has a significant impact on mortality rates. The null hypothesis that all the coefficients are jointly equal to zero was rejected for all but the two elderly black cohorts. However, examination of the individual coefficients yields little which is readily interpretable. The coefficients of HIND are positive in each of the male cohorts, as predicted. However, their magnitudes are small and only one of the four is statistically significant at the 90 percent confidence level. The two water system variables attain statistical significance four times, but the pattern of signs is inconsistent. The variable measuring suspended particulates also has very small coefficients and is insignificant in all eight cohorts. This is somewhat surprising, given the findings of Lave and Seskin and others.[11] However, this may be due to differences in the unit of observation and model specification.[12]

Finally, two of three climate variables seem to enter in a reasonably consistent manner: RAIN is positive and significant in four equations, and MJT is negative and significant in three equations. (SUN is also negative and significant in one equation.) These coefficients seem to be consistent with the traditional belief that cold and damp climates are bad for one's health. At the same time, however, these variables may be correlated with the geographic distribution of healthy people.[13] In particular, if it is relatively easier for healthy people to migrate to warmer and drier climates, which seems plausible for both economic and physical reasons, then these weather variables will reflect the impact of initial health on mortality, rather than the effects of climate. Unfortunately, these two interpretations cannot be distinguished with these data.

In general, the attempt to identify the impact of environmental factors on mortality rates has not been overly successful. If one is to use the health production function approach, then better data are needed in order to measure the relevant characteristics of air and water quality. Further-

TABLE 14

Coefficients of Environmental Variables, Deaths from Natural Causes, by Cohort

Cohort (N)	Environmental Variables						
	HIND	PWS	PSC	SUN	RAIN	MJT	PARTS
White males, 45-64 (286)	.0015†	.0034*	NS	.0014	.0045*	.0006	.0001
Black males, 45-64 (168)	.0005	-.0072**	.0056	-.0010	.0057*	.0021	.0004
White males, 65+ (286)	.0014	-.0003	.0001	-.0001	.0021*	-.0020*	NS
Black males, 65+ (116)	.0007	.0024	.0005	-.0055	-.0008	.0006	.0005
White females, 45-64 (286)	NA	.0036*	-.0021**	-.0027**	-.0007	-.0020*	NS
Black females, 45-64 (157)	NA	-.0029	.0029	.0010	.0070*	.0020	-.0001
White females, 65+ (286)	NA	.0002	-.0013	-.0011	.0004	-.0025*	NS
Black females, 65+ (123)	NA	.0022	-.0006	.0012	.0030	-.0038	NS

*Significant at 99 percent confidence level.
**Significant at 95 percent confidence level.
†Significant at 90 percent confidence level.
NA Not applicable.
NS Less than .00005.

more, variables should be constructed with data from several measuring stations within an area, so that meaningful values for an entire county, SMSA, or county group can be obtained.

Summary

The principal results of these analyses can be summarized straightforwardly. First, medical care use does appear to have a significant inverse relationship with age-sex-race-specific mortality rates from all causes of death. The elasticity of the mortality rate (from all causes) with respect to medical care is approximately -0.15 across all cohorts except the two middle-aged male cohorts. This means that an increase in medical care expenditures per capita of 10 percent would reduce mortality rates by about 1.5 percent. For white males, 45 to 64, the estimated decrease was larger, about -3.0 percent, and for black males, 45 to 64, it was smaller, about -0.8 percent.

Examination of medical care's coefficients in the cause-specific mortality analysis reinforces the basic finding. Its impact was generally insignificant in explaining variations in mortality rates from cancers and external causes. However, its coefficients were generally larger in magnitude in the equations for deaths from cardiovascular and ischemic heart disease than in the equations for deaths from all causes and from all natural causes.

This pattern is quite consistent with expectations based on changes in cause-specific mortality rates over time. Between 1960 and 1970, constant-dollar medical care expenditures increased by 82 percent. Over this same period, age-adjusted mortality rates (for all sexes and races) from cardiovascular diseases decreased by 14.8 percent. However, rates for deaths from cancer and accidents actually increased slightly, by 3.3 and 7.6 percent respectively. Since 1970, the mortality rate from accidents has reversed its trend and decreased by almost 20 percent. This may very well be the result of a concentrated effort, begun in the late 1960s by the federal government, to improve the quality and availability of emergency medical services, as well as of changes in automobile and highway design and of lower highway speed limits. Death rates from cancer have remained essentially unchanged, while the cardiovascular mortality rate has continued to decrease.

The findings with respect to other variables also generally conformed with prior expectations. The coefficients of several variables used as proxies for health status suggested that mortality rates are indeed higher where health is poorer. In addition, the implications of most of the lifestyle/behavior variables were consistent with prior findings in the literature. Marital status (percentage married), education, family income, and agricultural employment generally had negative associations with mortality rates.

Two indirect measures of alcohol and cigarette consumption had positive and statistically significant coefficients. The use of cigarettes sold per capita in the state as a proxy for actual consumption was reinforced by this variable's coefficients in the cause-specific mortality analysis. In particular, the coefficients were usually largest in magnitude, positive, and statistically significant in the ischemic heart and cardiovascular disease equations (for all but two cohorts—elderly females). Conversely, all coefficients but one were statistically insignificant in the equation for deaths from external causes. The coefficients in the cancer equations were positive for all four male cohorts, and statistically significant and larger in magnitude for the two middle-aged cohorts. However, none of the cigarette variable's coefficients were statistically significant in the equations for females.

Finally, analysis of the impact of environmental factors was limited by the lack of good quality data. Although the full set of environmental variables was generally significant as a group, interpretation of specific variables was difficult because of possible correlations with other factors. Accurate measurements of better defined variables for smaller geographic areas is needed for this type of study.

6

HEALTH PRODUCTION FUNCTION ESTIMATES: INFANT COHORTS

The basic theoretical model underlying the analysis of infant mortality rates is similar to that used in the analysis of adult mortality—mortality rates are a function of initial health, behavior, social and environmental conditions, and medical care. Following the successful results of studies by Phillips and Williams, and Williams,[1] factors other than medical care will be summarized by a set of variables which attempt to capture mortality risk at birth. The primary risk variable is the expected mortality rate, which is a function of the distribution of births by weight in each county group.

The great majority of infant deaths occur within the first 27 days of life, the neonatal period. Furthermore, the distribution of deaths by cause during this period is significantly different from that of the postneonatal period. Thus, infant deaths are partitioned into two sets, neonatal (1 to 27 days) and postneonatal (28 to 364 days). As with the adult cohorts, separate equations are estimated for each sex-race combination. Prenatal deaths will not be analyzed because the data on their frequency are much less reliable than those for infant deaths.

Medical care use is measured in two ways. As in the analysis of adult mortality, the first approach assumes that expenditures for prenatal, obstetric, and infant medical care are a constant proportion (across areas) of Medicare expenditures per enrollee. This permits the use of Medicare expenditures per enrollee as a measure of medical care use by the infant cohorts in the health production function. The second approach focuses on the availability of physicians who provide services to infants and pregnant women—obstetricians in the case of neonatal mortality and pediatricians for postneonatal mortality.

Finally, following the recent pathbreaking work of Grossman and Jacobowitz, we will investigate the impact of two major social programs: Medicaid and the liberalization of abortion laws.[2] This part of the analysis must be treated as exploratory, however, because of the crude ways in which the relevant variables are measured.

Empirical Specifications

1. DEPENDENT VARIABLES

As noted, there are three primary dependent variables: the infant mortality rate and its two components, the neonatal and postneonatal mortality rates. Rates are defined as the number of deaths per 1000 live births. Separate rates are computed by sex and race for each of the three variables.

Data on both births and deaths by age, sex, and race at the county level were obtained from the National Center for Health Statistics for the years 1969 to 1973.[3] County data were aggregated to the county group level and mortality rates computed by pooling data for the five-year period. This was done in order to smooth out the effects of random year-to-year fluctuations in births and deaths. In order to increase the reliability of the data, subsequent analyses are limited to county groups with at least 20 infant deaths per year in the relevant sex-race group. This results in 113 county groups for the analysis of black infant mortality and 387 county groups for the analysis of white infant mortality. Table 15 reports the means of the dependent variables. As is well known, rates for whites are

TABLE 15

AVERAGE INFANT MORTALITY RATES BY SEX, RACE, AND AGE AT DEATH,
COUNTY GROUPS, 1969–1973[a]
(DEATHS PER 1,000 LIVE BIRTHS, STANDARD DEVIATIONS IN PARENTHESES)

	NEONATAL	POSTNEONATAL	INFANT
Whites (387 county groups)			
Males	16.1(2.3)	4.6(1.2)	19.7(2.5)
Females	12.1(2.0)	3.7(1.0)	15.0(2.0)
Blacks (113 county groups)			
Males	26.2(4.3)	12.1(3.9)	35.0(4.9)
Females	20.8(4.2)	10.1(3.4)	28.8(3.9)

a. Unweighted county group means.

lower than those for blacks, and rates for females lower than those for males.

2. RISK VARIABLES

Numerous studies have shown that the single most important factor associated with infant mortality is weight at birth.[4] Following Phillips and Williams, and Williams,[5] an expected mortality rate is computed by multiplying age-sex-race-weight-specific mortality rates and each county group's distribution of births by weight. This relationship is represented by equation (6.1), where

$$EM_{jk} = \sum_{i=1}^{n} D_{ik}N_{ijk} \qquad k = 1,\ldots,4 \text{ sex and race combinations.} \quad (6.1)$$

EM_{jk} is the expected mortality rate for the jth county group and kth sex-race group, D_{ik} is the national mortality rate by sex and race for the ith birth-weight class, and N_{ijk} is the fraction of births in the ith birth-weight class by sex and race for the jth area.

Mortality rates by age, sex, race, and weight were obtained from a nationwide study of linked death and birth certificates for 107,038 infants who were born in 1960 and died before age 1.[6] Nine birthweight intervals were used in the computation (less than 1,000 grams up to 4,501 grams or more, in 500 gram intervals). In effect, this procedure creates a single variable which captures the effects of interarea variations in birthweight distributions and of age-sex-race differences in weight-specific mortality rates. The first component represents the generally unobservable effects on risk of variations in sociodemographic, environmental, and behavioral factors, while the second measures the probability of dying for each birth-weight class.

Two other measures of mortality risk at birth are the mother's age and the place of birth (in or out of hospital). Although its impact on mortality is less dramatic than that of birthweight, the mother's age has been consistently linked with mortality risk.[7] This factor will be measured by the percentage of births to young (less than 15) and old (35 or more) mothers.

Evidence regarding the impact of place of birth on mortality is more scanty. Kessner et al. used the type of hospital service as a factor in the index of adequacy of medical care (which was significantly related to infant mortality).[8] It will be assumed here that births outside of hospitals are more risky because of the absence of immediately available back-up medical care. Clearly, this variable differs from the other two risk factors in that it is not a measure of biological risk. As such, it may also be interpreted as a proxy for access to and use of medical care. (The variable reported in the results below is measured as the percentage of births in hospitals, for each sex-race group.)

Table 16 reports the means and standard deviations of the risk variables. Sex and race differences among the expected mortality rates follow the same pattern as the observed mortality rates. The expected rates are generally higher than the actual rates primarily because the expected mortality rates are based on 1960 age-sex-race-weight-specific mortality rates. Since 1960, there has been a continuing secular decline in mortality rates. Racial differences are also apparent in the other risk variables. Fewer than 7 percent of white births occur to mothers in high-risk age groups, while about 8 percent of black births occur to high-risk mothers. Similarly, almost all white births are in hospitals. The mean percentage of black births in hospitals is also quite high, almost 96 percent, but has a high standard deviation of about 7 percent.

3. MEDICAL CARE VARIABLES

Medical care consumption is measured in two ways. The first approach assumes that spending for prenatal, obstetric, and infant medical care services is a constant proportion of Medicare expenditures per enrollee in each county group. As is shown in Appendix A, the coefficient of this variable is an unbiased estimate of the coefficient of the true expenditure variable under the assumption that the mortality equation can be represented by a Cobb-Douglas production function.

The second approach assumes that spending for medical care is closely related to the stocks of physicians who provide the bulk of care to infants and pregnant women, that is, pediatricians and obstetricians. Phillips and Williams successfully used the number of obstetricians per 1,000 live births in their analysis of neonatal mortality.[9] By contrast, Grossman and Jacobowitz used a much more gross measure, active nonfederal physicians per 1,000 population, and obtained consistently positive coefficients for the effect of medical care on neonatal mortality.[10] Consequently, medical care will be measured by active nonfederal obstetricians per 1,000 live births in the neonatal mortality equations, and by active nonfederal pediatricians per 1,000 births in the postneonatal equations. Since infant mortality is the sum of neonatal and postneonatal mortality, medical care will be measured by the number of obstetricians and pediatricians per 1,000 births in the infant mortality equation.

Three additional variables are used with the physician stock measures as crude proxies for the quality of medical care. These are the proportion

TABLE 16

Mean Values of Risk Variables for Infant Mortalities by Sex and Race[a]
(standard deviations in parentheses)

	White Males (n = 387)	Black Males (n = 113)	White Females (n = 387)	Black Females (n = 113)
Expected Mortality Rates (per 1,000 live births)				
Neonatal	18.8(1.8)	31.6(4.0)	14.3(1.6)	24.9(3.4)
Postneonatal	6.6(0.2)	18.3(0.6)	5.1(0.2)	14.8(0.5)
Infant	25.3(2.0)	49.9(4.6)	19.4(1.8)	39.7(3.9)
Percentage of Births to Mothers of High-Risk Ages (PBHRM)	6.7(9.8)	7.9(1.5)	6.8(10.0)	8.0(1.6)
Percentage of Births in Hospitals (PBIH)	99.7(1.1)	95.7(6.9)	99.7(1.1)	95.5(7.2)

a. Unweighted county group means.

of active physicians over age 65, the proportion of active physicians who are not board certified, and the proportion of hospitals with intensive care nurseries. The first two variables are defined for the appropriate physician specialties in each mortality equation. Both are hypothesized to be postively related to mortality rates, while the proportion of hospitals with intensive care nurseries is expected to have a negative effect on mortality.

4. SOCIAL POLICY VARIABLES[11]

Grossman and Jacobowitz have investigated the effects of various social policies and programs on neonatal mortality rates across counties. Their analysis examined four programs: coverage of first-time pregnancies by Medicaid; maternal and infant care projects; the use of family planning clinics by low-income women; and changes in abortion laws. Their principal conclusion was that liberalization of abortion laws, which began in 1967 and became national policy in 1973 when the Supreme Court ruled restrictive abortion laws unconstitutional, was the single most important social policy change that has contributed to declining neonatal mortality.

This analysis will examine two of these areas: Medicaid coverage of unborn children and abortion reform. Differences in the unit of analysis (the county group rather than the county) make analysis of maternal and infant care programs and family planning clinics suspect, since these facilities are likely to serve clients who live nearby. In many cases, the county group is too large a geographic area to permit plausible analysis. A second problem arises because Medicaid programs and abortion laws apply to states, while some county groups cross state lines. Therefore, the analysis of these latter two policies will be limited to county groups which are wholly contained within a single state and which meet the criterion of at least 20 infant deaths per year in a sex-race cohort. Applying these screens reduces the number of county groups available for analysis to 304 for whites and 92 for blacks. Finally, the analysis will be conducted only for neonatal mortality rates, since these programs are likely to have their greatest effects during the neonatal period.

Medicaid programs differ widely in their rules for coverage of unborn children. Some states cover all pregnancies of Medicaid-eligible women, others cover pregnancies only if the father is not present (or in some states present but unemployed), while at the other extreme, 19 Medicaid programs do not cover any unborn children.[12] Because of this variation, Medicaid coverage will be measured by its complement, NOMCAID, which is defined as a dichotomous variable which takes the value 1 if the state program does not cover unborn children, and 0 otherwise. This variable is expected to have a positive impact on neonatal mortality.

The process of liberalizing abortion laws began in 1967 and culminated in the 1973 Supreme Court decision which found restrictive abortion laws unconstitutional. Systematic reporting of data on the number of abortions performed began only in 1971.[13] However, these data may not be very reliable as measures of all abortions for three reasons: illegal abortions are not included; the Center for Disease Control, which compiled the data, relies on reports from individual states, which differ in the completeness and methods of obtaining data; and about 10 percent of reported abortions cannot be allocated to a particular state because the woman's state of residence is not known. Because of these difficulties and in order to maintain comparability with Grossman and Jacobowitz, two abortion reform variables are created. One is a dichotomous variable which takes the value of 1 if the state liberalized its abortion law between 1967 and 1970, and takes the value 0 otherwise. The second is the number of abortions per 1,000 live births in each state between 1971 and 1973.[14] Table 17 summarizes the information on Medicaid coverage of unborn children, abortion law liberalization, and abortion rates by state. Because of the

TABLE 17

ABORTION RATES, ABORTION LAW LIBERALIZATION, AND MEDICAID COVERAGE
OF FIRST-TIME PREGNANCIES BY STATE, VARIOUS YEARS

STATE	ABORTIONS PER 1,000 LIVE BIRTHS 1973	YEAR ABORTION LAW LIBERALIZED (1970 OR EARLIER)	MEDICAID COVERAGE OF FIRST-TIME PREGNANCIES*
Alabama	33.2	—	2
Alaska	167.8	1970	0
Arizona	47.9	—	0
Arkansas	43.1	1969	0
California	352.7	1967	1
Colorado	153.3	1967	3
Connecticut	208.3	—	0
Delaware	223.7	1969	3
District of Columbia	788.6	—	3
Florida	116.5	—	0
Georgia	88.3	1968	0
Hawaii	286.1	1970	1
Idaho	25.3	—	0
Illinois	82.8	—	0
Indiana	58.7	—	0
Iowa	80.8	—	0
Kansas	137.3	1970	3
Kentucky	41.7	—	3
Louisiana	15.6	—	2
Maine	86.9	—	0
Maryland	228.4	1968	3
Massachusetts	222.7	—	1
Michigan	80.9	—	0
Minnesota	63.4	—	1
Mississippi	16.1	—	0
Missouri	91.2	—	0
Montana	27.2	—	3
Nebraska	68.9	—	3
Nevada	144.4	—	2
New Hampshire	112.9	—	0
New Jersey	240.3	—	0
New Mexico	147.4	1969	2
New York	421.6	1970	1
North Carolina	113.1	1967	0
North Dakota	23.6	—	2
Ohio	82.2	—	3
Oklahoma	49.9	—	0
Oregon	224.2	1969	3
Pennsylvania	88.8	—	1

TABLE 17 (cont'd)

ABORTION RATES, ABORTION LAW LIBERALIZATION, AND MEDICAID COVERAGE
OF FIRST-TIME PREGNANCIES BY STATE, VARIOUS YEARS

STATE	ABORTIONS PER 1,000 LIVE BIRTHS 1973	YEAR ABORTION LAW LIBERALIZED (1970 OR EARLIER)	MEDICAID COVERAGE OF FIRST-TIME PREGNANCIES*
Rhode Island	153.8	—	2
South Carolina	57.1	1970	2
South Dakota	33.7	—	2
Tennessee	59.7	—	2
Texas	54.7	—	0
Utah	18.4	—	1
Vermont	146.0	—	1
Virginia	130.8	1970	2
Washington	310.2	1970	1
West Virginia	31.2	—	3
Wisconsin	76.9	—	1
Wyoming	40.7	—	0

SOURCES: Abortions—U.S. Department of Health, Education and Welfare, Center for
Disease Control, *Abortion Surveillance: Annual Summaries for 1971, 1972,
and 1973.* Live Births—U.S. Department of Commerce, Bureau of the Census,
Statistical Abstract of the U.S., 1975, p. 55.
*0 = No coverage of first-time pregnancies.
  1 = Coverage of first-time pregnancies.
  2 = Covers first-time pregnancies only if father not present.
  3 = Covers first-time pregnancies if father not present or unemployed.

crude ways in which these variables are defined and measured, the results
reported should be regarded as exploratory and tentative.

Table 18 reports the means and standard deviations of the medical care
and social policy variables. Both sets are based on data for the county
group or state. Thus, differences between whites and blacks reflect differences in the geographic areas included in the calculations.

Results

This section is divided into two parts. The first focuses on the effects of
risk at birth and medical care on the three infant mortality measures:
neonatal, postneonatal, and infant mortality rates. The interrelationship
between medical care use and mortality risk is also explored. The sec-

TABLE 18

MEAN VALUES OF INDEPENDENT VARIABLES, INFANT MORTALITY EQUATIONS[a]
(STANDARD DEVIATIONS IN PARENTHESES)

VARIABLES	SYMBOL	WHITES (n = 387)	BLACKS (n = 113)
A. Medical Care Variables			
Medicare expenditures per enrollee ($)	MCDREXP	302.5(66.6)	305.2(85.9)
Pediatricians per 1,000 live births	PDPTB	4.1(3.3)	5.2(3.9)
Percentage pediatricians 65 and older	PPDOLD	5.9(6.4)	5.6(5.1)
Percentage pediatricians without board certification	PNBPDS	37.3(15.9)	44.9(14.1)
Obstetricians per 1,000 live births	OBPTB	4.6(2.9)	5.6(3.7)
Percentage obstetricians 65 and older	POBOLD	7.4(6.1)	7.9(5.2)
Percentage obstetricians without board certification	PNBOBS	38.6(13.6)	43.6(11.2)
Percentage hospitals with intensive care nurseries	PPNURS	41.5(21.5)	42.4(18.1)
B. Social Policy Variables[b]		(n = 304)	(n = 92)
State liberalized abortion law before 1971	ABLAW	0.3(0.5)	0.8(0.4)
Abortions per 1,000 live births	ABRATE	108.3(2.2)	103.1(5.8)
State Medicaid program does not cover unborn children	NOMCAID	0.4(0.5)	0.4(0.5)

a. Unweighted county group means.
b. County groups which cross state borders are excluded.

ond part examines the impacts of abortion liberalization and Medicaid coverage of unborn children on neonatal mortality rates.

All coefficients reported were estimated by ordinary least squares regression analysis. This method is appropriate because all of the independent variables are either exogenous or predetermined. Following the methods developed in the analysis of adult mortality rates, the estimating

equations are assumed to take a multiplicative (Cobb-Douglas) form in the key variables, medical care and expected mortality.
This form can be represented by

$$Y = AX_1^{\beta_1}X_2^{\beta_2}e^{(\Sigma\gamma_i Z_i)}U \qquad (6.2)$$

where

Y = observed mortality
X_1 = expected mortality
X_2 = medical care
Z_i = other independent variables
U = random error term
A = constant term.

1. RISK AT BIRTH AND MEDICAL CARE

Tables 19-21 present the regression coefficients for the basic health production model. Separate results are reported by sex, race, and age at death. Five specifications were estimated for each cohort and dependent variable. Specifications 1 and 3 include only two independent variables, the expected mortality rate and a medical care measure—Medicare expenditures per enrollee in specification 1 and active obstetricians and/or pediatricians per 1,000 live births in specification 3. Equations 2 and 4 add two additional risk factors, the percentage of births to mothers of high-risk age and the percentage of births in hospitals. Finally, the fifth specification adds three crude proxies for the quality of medical care, the percentage of obstetricians and/or pediatricians age 65 and older, the percentage without board certification, and the percentage of hospitals with intensive care nurseries.

The results for the white cohorts, both male and female, can be summarized readily. First, the expected mortality rate, which reflects variations in the distribution of births by weight, is clearly the most important factor explaining variations in mortality rates. It is consistently positive and highly significant in all specifications. Second, medical care, whether measured by Medicare expenditures per enrollee or physicians per 1,000 births, is consistently negative and statistically significant at the 99 percent confidence level in all specifications. Furthermore, the coefficients of the medical care variables are very stable across specifications, sex, and age at death. The coefficients imply that a 10 percent increase in medical care expenditures will reduce mortality rates by between 1.5 and 2 percent. Increasing the number of obstetricians and pediatricians per 1,000 live births by 10 percent would reduce mortality rates by about half as much, approximately 0.6 to 0.8 percent.[15]

TABLE 19
REGRESSION COEFFICIENTS—NEONATAL MORTALITY RATES

WHITES (n = 385)

	Males					Females				
	1	2	3	4	5	1	2	3	4	5
LENR[a]	.635*	.613*	.697*	.649*	.636*	.510*	.501*	.547*	.526*	.534*
PBHRM[a]		.146**		.239*	.202*		.079		.176*	.141**
PBIH[a]		-.644		-.161	-.286		NS		.498	.407
LMDCREXP	-.149*	-.140*				-.148*	-.144*			
LOBPTB			-.075*	-.080*	-.074*			-.075*	-.081*	-.076*
POLDOBS					.003*					.001**
PNBOBS					.001*					.001
PPNURS					NS					NS
Constant	1.700	2.345	.769	1.063	1.164	1.914	1.911	1.074	.627	.651
R² (adj)	.258	.267	.313	.338	.371	.198	.199	.247	.259	.270
F	67.828	36.026	88.663	50.029	33.288	48.441	32.785	63.880	34.488	21.257

BLACKS (n = 113)

	Males					Females				
	1	2	3	4	5	1	2	3	4	5
LENR[a]	.510*	.671*	.551*	.666*	.645*	.523*	.621*	.556*	.618*	.612*
PBHRM[a]		2.069†		2.046†	2.595**		1.047		1.071	1.159
PBIH[a]		-.317**		-.350	-.289		-.305		-.343	-.326
LMDCREXP	-.084	.031				-.079	-.035			
LOBPTB			-.045**	-.003	-.008			-.034	-.002	-.002
POLDOBS					-.003					.001
PNBOBS					-.002					-.001
PPNURS					.001†					NS
Constant	1.889	1.173	1.340	1.050	1.081	1.730	1.373	1.225	1.221	1.259
R² (adj)	.137	.189	.149	.187	.226	1.93	.216	.194	.213	.197
F	9.784	7.513	10.714	7.423	5.676	14.309	8.735	14.334	8.591	4.928

a. Sex-race-specific values.
*Significant at 99 percent confidence level.
**Significant at 95 percent confidence level.
†Significant at 90 percent confidence level.
NS Less than .0005.

Key:
LENR—Log expected neonatal mortality rate.
PBHRM—Percentage births to high-risk mothers.
PBIH—Percentage births in hospitals.
LMDCREXP—Log Medicare expenditures per enrollee.

LOBPTB—Log active obstetricians per 1,000 births.
POLDOBS—Percentage obstetricians 65 and older.
PNBOBS—Percentage obstetricians with no boards.
PPNURS—Percentage hospitals with intensive care nurseries.

TABLE 20
REGRESSION COEFFICIENTS—POSTNEONATAL MORTALITY RATES

WHITES (n = 385)

	Males					Females				
	1	2	3	4	5	1	2	3	4	5
LEPR[a]	1.162*	1.352*	1.437*	1.545*	1.640*	1.251*	1.310*	1.380*	1.378*	1.508*
PBHRM[a]		-.187†		-.115*	-.132		-.091*		-.011*	.008
PBIH[a]		-3.887		-3.531	-3.677**		-3.452		-3.261	-3.547*
LMDCREXP	-.145*	-.144*				-.198*	-.193*			
LPDPTB			-.075*	-.068*	-.063*			-.057*	-.050*	-.036**
POLDPDS					.002					-.001
PNBPDS					NS					-.001
PPNURS					-.001*					-.001*
Constant	.130	3.654	-1.129	2.185	2.208	.343	3.666	-.928	2.317	2.467
R² (adj)	.050	.093	.091	.122	.144	.064	.093	.061	.084	.097
F	11.106	10.799	20.277	14.298	10.219	14.214	10.837	13.540	9.807	6.910

BLACKS (n = 113)

	Males					Females				
	1	2	3	4	5	1	2	3	4	5
LEPR[a]	-1.417**	1.786**	-.288	1.871*	1.703*	-1.435†	.723	-.317	1.169	1.307
PBHRM[a]		.869		-.962	-1.186		-1.685		-4.072**	-5.014**
PBIH[a]		-2.651*		-2.449*	-2.524*		-2.201*		-2.314*	-2.268*
LMDCREXP	-.380*	-.173*				-.468*	-.310*			
LPDPTB			-.187*	-.111*	-.125*			-.187*	-.150*	-.150**
POLDPDS					.006†					-.006
PNBPDS					.001*					NS
PPNURS					NS					-.002†
Constant	8.636	.667	3.442	-.513	-.022	8.716	4.239	3.296	1.604	1.496
R² (adj)	.201	.481	.339	5.25	.532	.224	.357	.269	.388	.400
F	14.956	26.918	29.520	32.037	19.182	16.981	16.517	21.416	18.754	11.667

*Significant at 99 percent confidence level.
**Significant at 95 percent confidence level.
†Significant at 90 percent confidence level.
NS Less than .0005.
a. Sex-race-specific values.

Key:
LEPR—Log expected postneonatal mortality rate.
PBHRM—Percentage births to high-risk mothers.
PBIH—Percentage births in hospitals.
LMDCREXP—Log Medicare expenditures per enrollee.

LPDPTB—Log active pediatricians per 1,000 births.
POLDPDS—Percentage pediatricians 65 and older.
PNBPDS—Percentage pediatricians with no boards.
PPNURS—Percentage hospitals with intensive care nurseries.

TABLE 21
REGRESSION COEFFICIENTS—INFANT MORTALITY RATES

WHITES (n = 385)

	MALES					FEMALES				
	1	2	3	4	5	1	2	3	4	5
LEIR[a]	.661*		.744*	.717*	.713*	.566*	.565*	.616*	.601*	.606*
PBHRM[a]		.666*		.160*	.122**		.035		.128**	.094
PBIH[a]		-1.473*		-1.015**	-1.093**		-.996†		-.526	-.586*
LMDCREXP		-.140*					-.154*			
LDOCS	-.149*		-.078*	-.078*	-.076*	-.159*		-.077*	-.078*	-.076*
POLDDOCS					.191†					1.66
PNBDOCS					.109**					-.096**
PPNURS					-.001*					-.001†
Constant	1.685	3.081	.721	1.809	1.869	1.928	2.891	1.025	1.589	1.606
R² (adj)	.231	.245	.318	.336	.358	.207	.210	.275	.282	.295
F	58.666	32.217	90.354	49.543	31.528	51.021	26.588	73.922	38.795	23.943

BLACKS (n = 113)

	MALES					FEMALES				
	1	2	3	4	5	1	2	3	4	5
LEIR[a]	.305**	.749*	.478*	.760*	.721*	.282**	.569*	.435*	.617*	.641*
PBHRM[a]		1.262**		.491	.849†		-.024		-.853	-1.109
PBIH[a]		-1.074*		-.980*	-.981*		-.921*		-.889*	-.950*
LMDCREXP	-.182*	-.081†				-.204*	-.122**			
LDOCS			-.105*	-.055*	-.049**			-.094*	-.062*	-.057**
POLDDOCS					.099					.459
PNBDOCS					-.137**					-.107
PPNURS					-.001†					-.001
Constant	3.390	2.007	1.903	1.594	1.718	3.473	2.839	1.952	2.132	2.164
R² (adj)	.102	.340	.238	.336	.389	.133	.273	.185	.284	.296
F	7.273	15.392	18.359	17.176	11.182	9.504	11.515	13.612	12.107	7.751

*Significant at 99 percent confidence level.
**Significant at 95 percent confidence level.
†Significant at 90 percent confidence level.
a. Sex-race-specific values.

Key:
LEIR—Log expected infant mortality rate.
PBHRM—Percentage births to high-risk mothers.
PBIH—Percentage births in hospitals.
LMDCREXP—Log Medicare expenditures per enrollee.
LDOCS—Log active pediatricians and obstetricians per 1,000 births.
POLDDOCS—Percentage pediatricians and obstetricians 65 and older.
PNBDOCS—Percentage pediatricians and obstetricians with no boards.
PPNURS—Percentage hospitals with intensive care nurseries.

The coefficients of the other risk variables, percentage of births to high-risk mothers (PBHRM) and percentage of births in hospitals (PBIH), are less stable. PBHRM is positive and statistically significant in the neonatal equations (table 19) but negative and also significant in the postneonatal period (table 20). The coefficients in the infant mortality equations (table 21) reflect the greater weights of neonatal deaths—they are positive but smaller in magnitude and statistically significant in only three of six specifications. This pattern suggests that white babies born to either very young or very old mothers are more likely to die during the neonatal period than babies born to mothers of other ages. However, those that survive the first month of life do not have higher mortality rates than other infants. In fact, the postneonatal rate may be artificially lower in areas with relatively high proportions of births to high-risk mothers because fewer infants survive the neonatal period.

The coefficients of PBIH are negative, as expected, in all but the female neonatal equations (table 19). However, its impact on neonatal mortality rates is not statistically significant. Its coefficients are much larger in magnitude and generally statistically significant, with values ranging from -.526 to -1.473 in the infant mortality equations, and from -3.261 to -3.887 in the postneonatal mortality equations. Although more than 99 percent of white babies were born in hospitals in 1970 (table 16), these coefficients suggest that the reduction in mortality resulting from bringing the approximately 25,000 babies born outside of hospitals into the hospital system might be substantial. If values from table 21 are used, bringing the percentage of births in hospitals up to 100 percent would reduce infant mortality rates by about 1 percent. Caution should be exercised, however, in applying this result in the 1980s because of substantial changes in attitudes and circumstances surrounding out-of-hospital births.

Finally, the three quality of care variables seem to add little to the overall results. Only the coefficients of PPNURS, the percentage of hospitals with intensive care nurseries, are consistently negative as expected, although they are not statistically significant in the neonatal equations. The magnitudes of the coefficients are extremely small, however. This suggests that the payoff from adding more intensive care nurseries is negligible. The physicians' characteristics variables also have coefficients which are generally small in magnitude. Furthermore, their signs, which were hypothesized to be positive, do not show a consistent pattern.

Results for the black cohorts are less clearcut than those for whites. Coefficients are less stable across types of mortality and appear to be very sensitive to equation specification. The most dramatic example of this is the change in sign and statistical significance of the coefficients of the expected postneonatal mortality rates in the specifications which add the model's other two risk variables. The coefficients switch from negative (and statistically significant in two cases—specifications 1 and 3) to positive (and statistically significant for males—specifications 2 and 4). Similarly, the coefficients of the medical care variables are reduced in magnitude by about half when the additional risk variables are added.

This type of sensitivity is usually a sign of multicollinearity. Following Kmenta,[16] PBHRM and PBIH were regressed against the other independent variables in specification 2. The percentage of births in hospitals was found to have a strong positive correlation with both the expected mortality rate and Medicare expenditures per enrollee. Simple correlation coefficients ranged from 0.45 to 0.62, and regression R^2s ranged from 0.35 to 0.45. The percentage of births to high-risk mothers also had a fairly strong negative correlation with Medicare expenditures ($\rho = -0.56$ and R^2s between 0.28 and 0.33).

Under these conditions, it is clear that omission of PBHRM and PBIH will bias the coefficients of the expected mortality and medical care variables. The other side of the dilemma, however, is that their inclusion reduces the reliability of the coefficient estimates. These caveats must be kept in mind in interpreting the results for the black cohorts.

Except for specifications 1 and 3 for postneonatal mortality (table 20) the model's primary risk variable, expected mortality, enters all equations with the expected positive sign and is generally statistically significant. Of the other two risk variables, the percentage of births in hospitals always has a negative coefficient and is statistically significant in the postneonatal and infant mortality equations. It is not significant in the neonatal equations. The percentage of births to mothers of high risk ages has a positive though generally insignificant effect on neonatal mortality. It is not statistically significant in the other equations, except for female postneonatal mortality, where it has the wrong sign.

As noted, the coefficients of both medical care variables are very sensitive to the inclusion of the risk variables and also vary dramatically across dependent variables. In specifications 1 and 3, for example, the postneonatal medical care coefficients are about five times larger than those in the neonatal equations. Because of multicollinearity and specification problems, it is probably the case that the coefficient estimates of the medical care variables in the specifications with and without the additional risk variables bracket the true values of the coefficients. If it is arbitrarily assumed that the true values are the averages of the estimated bracket values, then it appears that medical care does have a negative impact on black mortality rates. Furthermore, the impact seems to be much larger on postneonatal than on neonatal rates. There is no clear reason for this result, although it may reflect the greater importance of risk factors on neonatal mortality.

Table 22 reports the average medical care coefficients. Note that the values in the black infant mortality equations are very similar to those estimated with data for whites. Also as in the equations for whites, the coefficients of Medicare expenditures per enrollee are consistently about twice as large as the coefficient of physicians (obstetricians and/or pediatricians) per 1,000 live births. Finally, the quality of care variables do not have any meaningful impact on the results. Only one coefficient is statistically significant (at the 90 percent confidence level) and several enter with the wrong sign.

The instability of the medical care coefficients in the regressions for blacks raises a more general concern about the basic specification reported here. If one of the ways medical care affects infant health is by reducing risk at birth, for example, through early and continuous prenatal care, then the impact of medical care may be understated in the above results because risk at birth is explicitly included in the equation specification. This issue is explored by estimating a simplified version of the health production function in two steps. The first step includes only medical care. On the second step, the expected mortality rate is added to the specification.

The results of this exercise are presented in table 23, which reports the medical care variables' coefficients by sex, race, and age at death. As can be readily seen, including both medical care and the expected mortality rate in the specifications generally has only a small impact on the magnitude of the medical care coefficients. Except for the equations for black neonatal mortality, the average change in a coefficient's magnitude is about 13 percent. It is also the case, more often than not, that the medical care coefficient is larger in absolute magnitude when the expected mortality rate is included in the equation than when it is omitted.

If one treats the specification with the expected mortality rate excluded as an equation with a relevant variable omitted, then it is possible to make an indirect inference about the aggregate relationship between the use of medical care and the expected mortality rate. It is well known that the coefficient of the included variable, medical care, will be unbiased only if $\beta_2 \rho_{12} = 0$, where β_2 is the coefficient of the omitted variable, the expected mortality rate, and ρ_{12} is the correlation between the expected mortality rate and the medical care variable. We know from tables 19–21 that β_2 is positive in sign and large in magnitude. Since the medical care coefficients change only slightly when the expected mortality rate is omitted (table 23),

TABLE 22

AVERAGE MEDICAL CARE COEFFICIENTS, BLACKS,
BY SEX AND AGE AT DEATH

| | MALES | | | FEMALES | | |
	Neonatal	Postneonatal	Infant	Neonatal	Postneonatal	Infant
LMDCREXP[a]	−.058	−.277	−.132	−.057	−.389	−.163
LOBPTB[b]	−.024			−.018		
LPDPTB[b]		−.149			−.169	
LDOCS[b]			−.080			−.078

a. The average of coefficient values from specifications 1 and 2, tables 19–21.
b. The average of coefficient values from specifications 3 and 4, tables 19–21.

TABLE 23

COEFFICIENTS FROM EQUATIONS WITH AND WITHOUT THE
EXPECTED MORTALITY RATE BY AGE AT DEATH, SEX, AND RACE

	Expected Mortality Excluded				Expected Mortality Included			
	White Males	White Females	Black Males	Black Females	White Males	White Females	Black Males	Black Females
Neonatal Mortality[a]								
LMDCREXP	−.167*	−.143*	−.010	−.003	−.149*	−.148*	−.084	−.079
LOBPTB	−.066*	−.064*	−.003	.018	−.075*	−.075*	−.045*	−.034
Postneonatal Mortality[a]								
LMDCREXP	−.134*	−.174*	−.430*	−.517*	−.146*	−.198*	−.380*	−.467*
LPDPTB	−.060*	−.041*	−.192*	−.193*	−.075*	−.057*	−.187*	−.187*
Infant Mortality[a]								
LMDCREXP	−.161*	−.151*	−.151*	−.175*	−.149*	−.159*	−.182*	−.204*
LDOCS	−.068*	−.066*	−.080*	−.068*	−.078*	−.077*	−.105*	−.094*

*Significant at the 99 percent confidence level.
a. Measured in natural logarithms.
Key: LMDCREXP—Log Medicare expenditures per enrollee.
LOBPTB—Log active obstetricians per 1,000 births.
LPDPTB—Log active pediatricians per 1,000 births.
LDOCS—Log active pediatricians and obstetricians per 1,000 births.

this implies that ρ_{12} is relatively small in magnitude. The fact that the medical care coefficients tend to be larger in absolute value (in 18 of 24 equations) when expected mortality is excluded suggests that ρ_{12} is typically positive.

One should be careful, however, not to confuse this aggregate cross-sectional relationship with results based on the observation of individual pregnancies over time. Numerous studies cited in chapter 3 have found that the application of early and continuous prenatal care has a positive effect on pregnancy outcomes. It does not follow, however, that the actual aggregate distribution of infant-health related resources across areas in 1970 was necessarily related to aggregate pregnancy outcomes. In fact, the relatively small impact on the medical care coefficients of adding the expected mortality rate suggests that the two were distributed relatively independently in the aggregate.

2. NEONATAL MORTALITY AND SOCIAL POLICY VARIABLES

In order to concentrate on the effects of Medicaid coverage of unborn children and abortion law liberalization, the model reported next contains only two other independent variables, the expected neonatal mortality rate and the number of obstetricians per 1,000 live births. (Medicare expenditures per enrollee were highly correlated with the abortion rate variable. As a result, coefficient estimates were unstable and unreliable.) Two specifications are reported for each sex-race group. One measures abortion law liberalization by a continuous variable, LABRATE, which is the log of the number of abortions per 1,000 live births in each state. (This variable is not measured separately by maternal race or age.) The second specification measures abortion liberalization by a dichotomous variable, ABLAW, which takes the value 1 if the state reformed its abortion law between 1967 and 1970. Medicaid coverage is measured by NOMCAID, a dichotomous variable which equals 1 if the state's Medicaid program does not cover unborn children.

Regression coefficients are reported in table 24. As in the previous section, the expected mortality rate has the largest impact and is consistently significant at the 99 percent confidence level. Similarly, medical care enters with consistently negative coefficients and is statistically significant in almost all specifications.

The coefficients of the social policy variables indicate that both Medicaid coverage of unborn children and abortion law liberalization contribute to reduced neonatal mortality rates. Medicaid coefficients are

TABLE 24
Neonatal Mortality and Social Policy Variables, Regression Coefficients by Race and Sex

	White Males (n = 304)						White Females (n = 304)				
	1	2	3	4	5		1	2	3	4	5
LENR	.65*	.63*	.65*	.62*	.64*		.48*	.50*	.49*	.49*	.48*
LOBPTB	-.06*	-.05*	-.06*	-.05*	-.06*		-.06*	-.05*	-.06*	-.05*	-.06*
NOMCAID	.05*			.04*	.04*		.04*			.03**	.03**
ABRATE		-.05*		-.04*				-.04*		-.04*	
ABLAW			-.03*		-.02				-.03**		-.02
R^2 (adj)	.29	.32	.28	.33	.30		.22	.25	.21	.26	.22

	Black Males (n = 92)						Black Females (n = 92)				
	1	2	3	4	5		1	2	3	4	5
LENR	.60*	.62*	.58*	.60*	.57*		.63*	.66*	.62*	.64*	.61*
LOBPTB	-.05**	-.05**	-.05**	-.05	-.05**		-.04	-.04	-.04	-.03	-.04
NOMCAID	.05			.05	.04		.03			.03	.02
ABRATE		-.01		-.01				-.01		-.01	
ABLAW			-.07**		-.06**				-.05†		-.05
R^2 (adj)	.21	.19	.24	.21	.24		.24	.23	.26	.23	.25

*Significant at 99 percent confidence level.　　ABRATE—Abortions per 1,000 births.
**Significant at 95 percent confidence level.　　ABLAW—Equals 1 if state liberalized its abortion law between 1967 and 1970; otherwise 0.
†Significant at 90 percent confidence level.
Key: LENR—Log expected neonatal mortality rate.
　　LOBPTB—Log active obstetricians per 1,000 births.
　　NOMCAID—Equals 1 if Medicaid program does not cover first-time pregnancies; otherwise 0.

fairly stable and slightly larger for males than for females; 0.04 or 0.05 for males and 0.02 or 0.03 for females. With the impact of medical care held constant, these coefficients imply that in states which do not cover unborn children, neonatal mortality rates are between 4 and 5 percent higher for males, and between 2 and 3 percent higher for females than in other states. These higher mortality rates are equivalent to roughly 28 more deaths per 100,000 white female births at one extreme, and to 107 more deaths per 100,000 black male births at the other extreme.

The implications of the abortion law variables are somewhat less clear, even though all coefficients show a negative effect on neonatal mortality rates. The coefficients of ABRATE indicate that abortion has had a larger effect on whites than on blacks. The coefficients of ABLAW, on the other hand, indicate the opposite—black neonatal rates were reduced more than white rates in states which reformed their abortion laws prior to 1971.

The ABRATE coefficients suggest that a 10 percent increase in abortion rates would reduce neonatal mortality rates from 1.9 deaths per 100,000 live births (black females) to 6.0 deaths per 100,000 live births (white males). Although the impact of the abortion rate variable appears small, it must be remembered that this is based on a 10 percent increase over a mean national rate in 1971–1973 of about 255 abortions per 1,000 live births. The coefficients also imply that reducing the abortion rate to its 1969 level of approximately 4 abortions per 1,000 live births would increase neonatal mortality rates by about 25 percent for whites and 6 percent for blacks. The estimated impact on whites is very similar to that reported by Grossman and Jacobowitz.[17] The impact on blacks is much smaller. This is very likely due to the crudeness of the data and to differences in model specification and units of analysis. The results reported here also differ from Grossman and Jacobowitz in that both medical care and Medicaid coverage of unborn children were found to have statistically significant effects.

Although these findings must be treated as exploratory, they do add another dimension to the debates over Medicaid coverage limits, federal financing of abortions, and constitutional bans against abortion. Namely, failure to cover unborn children under Medicaid and restrictions on abortions lead to subsequent increases in social costs through higher neonatal mortality rates. These costs take two forms: medical care expenditures for infants who die in the first month of life and the emotional impact on parents of babies who die. Although the latter cannot be readily measured, the former represents a possibly important area for further inquiry.

Summary

This chapter estimated a set of health production functions with various infant mortality rates as dependent variables. The basic model can be summarized succinctly—infant mortality is a function of risk at birth and medical care consumption. In addition, an exploratory analysis of the effects of two major social policies, Medicaid coverage of unborn children and abortion law liberalization, was also conducted. Separate equations were estimated for four sex-race cohorts and three ages of death, neonatal, postneonatal, and all deaths in the first year of life.

The principal results can be summarized readily. First, risk at birth is clearly the most important determinant of infant mortality. The expected mortality rate, a weighted measure of the distribution of births by birthweight, was statistically significant in almost all equations. The percentage of births in hospitals also had a large impact in the postneonatal and infant mortality equations. The percentage of births to mothers of high-risk age was generally less significant.

Second, increased medical care use also contributes to reduced mortality rates. The results were very strong for whites—an increase of 10 percent in medical care spending per capita would reduce mortality rates by about 1.5 percent. The results for blacks were less reliable because of greater multicollinearity and specification problems. However, the magnitude of the estimated impact of medical care was very similar to that for whites.

The negative relationship between medical care and mortality rates was observed for both approaches to measuring medical care use, that is, Medicare expenditures per enrollee and the numbers of active, patient care obstetricians and pediatricians per 1,000 live births. This is in sharp contrast to the analysis of adult mortality rates reported in chapter 4. There, it was found that the numbers of active patient care physicians per 1,000 population had typically no or implausible relationships with adult mortality rates. A possible explanation of these different findings may be that the services provided and patients treated by pediatricians and obstetricians are much more narrowly defined than those of all physicians treating a much larger and more diverse adult population. Consequently, the availability of pediatricians and obstetricians may be much more closely correlated with the actual use of medical care services geared toward reducing infant mortality rates than is the case for all patient care physicians' services and adult mortality rates. It also seems plausible that patients cross county-group borders less frequently for obstetrical and pediatric services than for adult medical services. This too would increase the correlation between the availability of pediatricians and obstetricians and the actual use of services.

It is also interesting to note that the coefficients of the Medicare expenditure variables are consistently twice as large as the coefficients of the pediatrician and obstetrician variables. This relationship implies that a given percentage increase in physician availability will increase per capita expenditures for medical care by about half as much, for example, a 10 percent increase in physicians per capita will increase medical care expenditures per capita by 5 percent. (In chapter 8, additional evidence which corroborates this inference will be presented.)

Finally, both of the social policies examined appear to have statistically significant effects on neonatal mortality rates. States which do not cover first-time pregnancies through their Medicaid programs have higher neonatal mortality rates than other states. Neonatal mortality rates were lower, however, in states which had relaxed their abortion laws before 1971 or had relatively higher abortion rates (abortions per 1,000 live births). Although these results must be considered tentative because of the crude way in which these variables were constructed, the mechanisms through which these policies influence neonatal mortality seem clear. Broader Medicaid coverage probably leads to earlier and more frequent prenatal care for eligible women. Abortion rates are higher for very young and very old women than for women of prime childbearing age, higher for single than for married women, and higher for blacks than for whites. Since each of these relationships is associated with greater risks at birth, higher abortion rates probably imply a smaller proportion of high-risk births.

Infant mortality rates have fallen dramatically since the late 1960s, by 38.6 percent between 1969 and 1978. Each of the factors analyzed in the infant mortality model has contributed to this decline. Table 25 reports percentage changes in some of the model's variables between 1969 and 1978. The largest changes occurred in the availability of medical care and the percentages of births to high-risk mothers. Changes were smaller for the other two variables, but these factors had larger quantitative impacts in the infant mortality equations. The only adverse movement was a slight decrease in the proportion of white babies born in hospitals.

How important have these factors been to the observed decline in infant mortality rates? Crude estimates of the relative importance of each variable can be made by combining the parameters reported in the infant mortality equations and the percentage changes in the explanatory variables.[18] As expected, the drop in the percentage of low birthweight babies had the largest impact of the four variables, accounting for almost 35 per-

TABLE 25

CHANGES IN FACTORS AFFECTING INFANT MORTALITY BY RACE, 1969-1978

	WHITES			BLACKS		
	1969	1978	Percentage Change	1969	1978	Percentage Change
Infant mortality[a]	19.0	12.7	−33.2	38.8	25.5	−34.3
Percentage low birthweight births[b]	7.1	5.9	−16.9	14.2	12.9	−9.2
Percentage births to high-risk mothers[c]	6.9	4.7	−31.9	8.1	5.2	−35.8
Percentage births in hospitals[d]	99.6	99.0	−0.7	95.9	99.0	3.2
Pediatricians per 1,000 live births[e,f]	3.8	6.3	66.0	3.8	6.3	66.0
Obstetricians per 1,000 live births[e,f]	4.3	6.5	50.6	4.3	6.5	50.6

SOURCES: HEW, National Center for Health Statistics, *Annual Natality and Mortality Statistics;* AMA, *Physician Distribution in The United States,* 1969 and 1977 editions.

a. Deaths per 1,000 live births; rate for blacks includes other nonwhite races.
b. Less than 2,500 grams.
c. Mothers younger than 15 or older than 34.
d. With physicians in attendance.
e. Active, nonfederal patient care physicians.
f. Data apply to all races.

cent of the decline in white infant mortality rates and 20 percent of the drop in black infant mortality rates. (These estimates probably understate the true impact of higher birthweights since no account is taken of the probable decreases in weight-specific mortality rates.) Medical care use, as measured by the availability of obstetricians and pediatricians per 1,000 live births, is the second most important factor, accounting for about 13 percent of the decrease in both black and white infant mortality rates. The medical care effect is even stronger for blacks if one interprets the percentage of births in hospitals as a joint measure of both access to medical care and risk at birth. In all, the four factors are responsible for between 38 to 47 percent of the drop in infant mortality rates.

This analysis strongly suggests that increased medical care use by pregnant women and infants leads to reduced infant mortality. Whether this is a "good" policy which should be continued depends on two factors: the value to society of saving an infant's life and the costs of other policies aimed at lowering infant mortality. The former is essentially a political question. The latter depends in large part on understanding the factors which influence the proportion of low birthweight babies. To date, little of use to formulating policy is known about this question.[19]

7

INCOME, EDUCATION, AND MORTALITY RATES

One of the more consistent findings of the earlier research on variations in mortality rates was that higher incomes and living standards are associated with lower mortality rates. Several more recent studies, however, have produced results which suggest an insignificant or possibly positive relationship between income and mortality rates.[1] Although the factors underlying the latter relationship are not well understood, several hypotheses have been offered to explain this apparent paradox. They include the existence of a ceiling, already reached by certain population groups, on the ability of standards of living to improve health; positive income-elasticities of demand for certain goods whose consumption adversely affects health; and the existence of certain nonconsumption factors, associated with higher-income occupations, which have deleterious health consequences (psychological pressure and tensions in managerial occupations, for example).

A better understanding of the income-mortality relationship may be particularly useful in this time of "budget crisis." With all levels of government concerned about the size and growth of transfer payments, which constitute a substantial portion of the incomes of certain population subgroups, it is important to ask what consequences cuts in transfer payments might have on the health of the population. Will mortality rates increase, decrease, level off, or remain unaffected with changes in income?

The primary objective of this chapter is to extend the earlier research in two important ways. First, income is decomposed into several components

---

Anthony Osei is the coauthor of this chapter.

in order to determine whether different types of income, that is, different ways of earning income, have differential effects on mortality rates. Second, separate analyses are conducted for each of the 12 population cohorts which were studied in the previous chapters. Since the mortality, income, education, and several other sociodemographic variables are all cohort-specific, these data are generally more accurate than those used in other studies of the income-mortality relationship. In addition, the analysis will explicity consider the potentially confounding effects on the parameter estimates caused by the close relationship between income and education.

Methods

The results reported for adults are based on the final specification of the mortality regressions with deaths from all causes as the dependent variable. (See table 9 for means of the dependent and independent variables for each adult cohort.) The results for infants, however, are based on a different specification from the one described in chapter 6, since the latter did not include income as an explicit variable. It was assumed that the effects of income and other sociodemographic, behavioral, and environmental factors operate through their impact on risk at birth. Therefore, the results for infants are based on an alternative specification which adds income, education, and several other variables to the model described in chapter 6.[2]

The mortality equations are estimated with several alternative definitions of income. The goal is to investigate whether the various components of income have different associations with mortality rates. The particular income variables used are as follows: total family income (TFI)—the sum of the dollar amounts of wages, salary income, net nonfarm and farm self-employment, and other income of all household members 14 years old and over; earned income (EI)—the sum of wages, salaries, commissions, bonuses or tips from all jobs and self-employment, professional, and farm income before deductions (excluding military bonuses, reimbursements, and pay in kind); unearned income (UI)—total family income less earned income (TFI-EI); Social Security income (SSI)—U.S. government payments to retired persons, to dependents of deceased insured workers, or to disabled workers (excluding Medicare reimbursements); welfare income (WI)—amounts received from federal, state, and local public programs such as AFDC, old age assistance, general assistance, and aid to the blind or totally disabled; transfer income (TI)—the sum of SSI and WI; and other unearned income (OUI)—interest, dividends, veterans' payments, retirement pensions from private employers, unions, and other governmental agencies, rental income, workman's compensation, alimony, private welfare payments, and contributions from persons not members of the household. Total family income (TFI) and unearned income (UI) are based on data for individuals' households; the other income variables are based only on individuals' incomes.

Table 26 reports the means of the income variables for each cohort. As is well known, whites have higher family incomes than blacks in each age-sex group, by factors ranging from 60 to 85 percent. White-black differences are much smaller for transfer incomes from public sources (Social Security payments and welfare income). In fact, blacks have higher levels of transfer income than whites except in the two elderly age groups. Differences are much greater, on the other hand, for transfer and unearned income from private sources (OUI), with whites having from two to six times more income from these sources than blacks.

Several earlier studies have emphasized the difficulty of untangling the effects of income on mortality rates from those of education.[3] This problem was addressed by estimating each mortality equation both with and without the education variable in order to gauge the strength of the interrelationship between these factors. In all, 14 specifications were estimated. The last seven are essentially the same as the first seven, except they exclude the education variable. The seven main specifications differ with respect to the definition of income: (1) total family income, (2) earned income and unearned income, (3) earned income, (4) unearned income, (5) transfer income, (6) Social Security income and welfare income, and, lastly, (7) other unearned income. (Specifications 2 and 6 include two separate income components.)

Results

The coefficients of the adult cohorts' income variables (from the equations with education included) are reported in table 27. Although the underlying equations explain exceedingly high proportions of the variance in mortality from all causes (R^2s vary around .9), these coefficients do not provide an unambiguous resolution of the income-mortality issue. The frequency of negative income coefficients appears to tilt the balance in favor of an inverse relationship, but a number of the coefficients are not statistically significant. In specification 1, for example, the coefficients of TFI, total family income, are negative for five of the cohorts but statistically significant only for the two middle-aged male cohorts.

TABLE 26
MEAN VALUES OF INCOME VARIABLES BY COHORT

	WHITE MALES, 45–64	WHITE MALES, 65+	BLACK MALES, 45–64	BLACK MALES, 65+	WHITE FEMALES, 45–64	WHITE FEMALES, 65+	BLACK FEMALES, 45–64	BLACK FEMALES, 65+	WHITE FEMALES, 14–44	BLACK FEMALES, 14–44
TFI-Total family income	$11,791	$6,570	$7,272	$3,941	$10,376	$5,863	$6,226	$3,811	$11,691	$6,821
EI-Earned income	8,242	1,638	4,377	857	2,060	405	1,559	303	1,971	2,012
UI-Unearned income	3,463	3,808	2,733	2,225	8,229	4,732	4,466	2,842	9,720	4,609
SSI-Social Security income	83	1,089	110	730	83	666	101	468	18	35
WI-Welfare income	3	35	52	129	4	59	99	198	16	130
TI-Transfer income	86	1,125	162	859	87	725	200	666	34	165
OUI-Other unearned income	603	1,327	143	268	265	673	627	113	104	39

Definitions:

Total family income—The sum of the dollar amounts of wages, salary income, net nonfarm and farm self-employment, and other income of *all* household members 14 years old and over.

Earned income—Includes wages, salaries, commissions, bonuses or tips from all jobs and self-employment, professional, and farm income before deductions (excluding military bonuses, reimbursement, and pay in kind).

Unearned income—Total family income less earned income.

Social Security income—Includes U.S. government payments to retired persons, to dependents of deceased insured workers, or to disabled workers (excluding Medicare reimbursements).

Welfare income—Includes amounts received from federal, state, and local public programs such as AFDC, old age assistance, general assistance, and aid to the blind or totally disabled.

Transfer income—The sum of Social Security income and welfare income.

Other unearned income—Includes interest, dividends, veterans payments, retirement pensions from private employers, unions, and other governmental agencies, rental income, workman's compensation, alimony, private welfare payments, and contributions from persons not members of the household.

TABLE 27

INCOME COEFFICIENTS, ADULT COHORTS
(EDUCATION INCLUDED)

INCOME SPECIFICATION	WHITE MALES, 45–64	WHITE MALES, 65+	BLACK MALES, 45–64	BLACK MALES, 65+	WHITE FEMALES, 45–64	WHITE FEMALES, 65+	BLACK FEMALES, 45–64	BLACK FEMALES, 65+
1 TFI	−.0006**	−.0003	−.0016*	.0003	−.0003	NS	.0003	−.0003
2 [UI	.0006	−.0010†	.0006	−.0009	.0001	.0005	.0001	−.0001
EI	−.0010*	.0007	−.0033*	.0032**	−.0032**	−.0095*	.0013	.0007
3 UI	.0003	−.0007†	−.0002	−.0005	−.0002	.0001	.0002	−.0003
4 EI	−.0010*	.0002	−.0032*	.0029**	−.0030**	−.0084*	.0014	.0007
5 TI	−.0106†	−.0021	.0060	−.0039	.0117†	.0195*	−.0031	−.0118**
6 [SSI	−.0073	.0009	.0143†	.0001	.0110†	.0283*	.0009	−.0009
WI	−.0272†	−.0247*	−.0087	−.0223*	.0158	−.0118	−.0058	−.0023*
7 OUI	−.0028†	−.0037†	−.0040	.0041†	−.0148*	−.0052*	−.0216**	−.0200*

*Significant at the 99 percent confidence level.
**Significant at the 95 percent confidence level.
†Significant at the 90 percent confidence level.
NS Less than .00005.

When total family income is decomposed into its earned (EI) and unearned (UI) components, a different pattern emerges. Earned income coefficients are negative and significant for three of four middle-aged cohorts and positive for three of four elderly cohorts. For unearned income however, the signs of the coefficients are reversed between middle-aged and elderly cohorts. In general, the pattern is that UI has a positive effect for the younger cohorts and a negative effect for elderly cohorts. This should not be too surprising, however, since this variable captures in part the influence of initial health, which affects both labor force participation and mortality rates. People in good health and of greater economic means generally have higher earned incomes while of working age, and higher unearned income (and thus less need to work) while of retirement age.

Specifications 3 and 4 estimate the impact of earned and unearned income separately. The results suggest no significant qualitative or quantitative differences from specification 2 on the impact of both EI and UI on mortality rates either through joint or independent estimation. The coefficients of both earned and unearned income are essentially identical to those estimated by specification 2.

The remaining specifications focus on different components of unearned income. As noted, UI includes the earnings of other family members as well as rental and capital income and various transfer payments from public and private sources. Looking first at public transfer programs, specification 5 examines the impact of transfer income. In general, the results are ambiguous. Although five of the coefficients are negative, only two are statistically significant. However, two of the three positive coefficients are also statistically significant. These results do not lend themselves to meaningful interpretation.

Decomposing public transfer payments into Social Security payments and welfare payments helps to clarify somewhat the ambiguity of the TI coefficients. In particular, seven of the eight coefficients of welfare income are negative, with four statistically significant. Conversely, six of the SSI coefficients have positive signs, with three statistically significant. Since SSI includes payments to the disabled and to the spouses of deceased insurees, who generally have higher mortality rates than either married or single people,[4] it may be that this variable is strongly associated with poor health status.

Finally, the last specification focuses on unearned income from capital sources and from private pension plans. The quantitative results for this variable are very similar to those for pure transfer payments, WI. The coefficients are negative for seven of the eight cohorts and five of these are also statistically significant. The strength of this finding may be due to the fact that this form of unearned income is the least likely to be related to health status. As such, it may be the best measure of economic status.

The results for the infant cohorts (from the specification including education) are presented in table 28. In general, the evidence suggests a fairly consistent negative relationship between mortality and income for all seven specifications. Coefficients are similar in magnitude for female and white male infants but generally smaller in magnitude for black male infants. Both mothers' earned income and unearned income from all sources, which consists primarily of spouse's and other family members' earnings, have uniformly negative signs and are statistically significant in all but one case. The impact of public transfer income, which is a very small component of total family income on average, is ambiguous. The coefficients of TI, SSI, and WI are generally insignificant. Finally, private transfer income, which makes up less than 1 percent of total income, has negative coefficients for three of the four cohorts.

As is well known, education and income are highly correlated. Thus, including an education variable in the regression equations increases the unreliability of the estimated income coefficients and makes their interpretation more ambiguous. Analysis of the simple correlation coefficients between TFI and education provides evidence to support this hypothesis.

TABLE 28

INCOME COEFFICIENTS, INFANT COHORTS
(EDUCATION INCLUDED)

INCOME SPECIFICATION		MALES		FEMALES	
		Blacks	Whites	Blacks	Whites
1	TFI	−.0007	−.0016*	−.0023**	−.0019*
2	UI	.0012	−.0011*	−.0014	−.0017*
	EI	−.0063†	−.0085*	−.0048	−.0043†
3	UI	−.0001	−.0014*	−.0024†	−.0019*
4	EI	−.0051†	−.0106*	−.0063†	−.0076*
5	TI	.0002	.0110	−.0036	.0015
6	SSI	−.0243	.0197†	−.0406†	.0068
	WI	.0114	.0008	.0128	−.0047
7	OUI	−.0093	−.0136†	.0142	−.0112†

*Significant at the 99 percent confidence level.
**Significant at the 95 percent confidence level.
†Significant at the 90 percent confidence level.

The correlation coefficients vary from .184 (elderly white males) to .766 (middle-aged white males) for the adult cohorts and .561 (blacks) to .770 (whites) for the infant cohorts (based on data for women of childbearing age). However, the apparent presence of a relatively high degree of multicollinearity is not sufficient reason to follow Silver and exclude education from our equations.[5] First, there is ample evidence in the literature to suggest the relevance of education as an important explanatory factor of mortality rates. Second, the exclusion of a relevant variable such as education may lead to serious error: not only will the estimated coefficients be biased, but inferences based on them will also be inaccurate. As Johnston suggests, "data and degrees of freedom permitting, one should err on the side of including variables in the regression analysis rather than excluding them."[6]

In order to gauge the impact of multicollinearity on the results, we also report the income coefficients from equations which exclude the education variable. These results are presented in tables 29 and 30. In general, the signs of the coefficients suggest an inverse relationship between income and mortality. As expected, most of the coefficients are negatively biased.[7] Only one coefficient (elderly black males) appears to have a positive bias. For total family income (TFI) the average increase in absolute value for the negative coefficients is about 50 percent.

A similar analysis of the effect of income on the education coefficients can be conducted by estimating regressions that include and exclude the income variables. The result of such an analysis for all cohorts is presented in table 31, where the income variable in question is total family income. As can be gleaned from the table, education coefficients with total family income excluded are in general negatively biased and larger in absolute value than those with family income included. Nine out of twelve coefficients increase in absolute value, on average by about 60 percent, with the maximum and minimum changes occurring for middle-aged white females and elderly black males, respectively. In general, education has a consistently negative association with mortality rates.

Summary

Several research and policy issues were raised at the outset of this chapter. Is income a significant factor in explaining geographic variations in adult mortality rates? What are the differential effects (if any) of the various components of income? What is the effect of 'pure' unearned income on mortality rates?

TABLE 29

INCOME COEFFICIENTS, ADULT COHORTS
(EDUCATION EXCLUDED)

INCOME SPECIFICATION		WHITE MALES, 45-64	WHITE MALES, 65+	BLACK MALES, 45-64	BLACK MALES, 65+	WHITE FEMALES, 45-64	WHITE FEMALES, 65+	BLACK FEMALES, 45-64	BLACK FEMALES, 65+
1	TFI	-.0011*	-.0003	-.0016*	-.0004	-.0002	-.0004†	NS	-.0005
2	[UI	.0005	-.0006**	.0009	-.0009	.0001	-.0003	.0002	-.0005
	EI	-.0017*	.0007	-.0034*	.0007	-.0026†	-.0034†	-.0004	-.0014
3	UI	-.0002	-.0005†	NS	-.0008	-.0001	-.0004†	.0001	-.0005
4	EI	-.0017*	.0002	-.0032*	.0004	-.0023†	-.0039†	-.0003	-.0016
5	TI	.0029	-.0033†	.0023	.0032	.0128**	.0126*	-.0057	-.0017
6	[SSI	.0075	-.0029	.0117†	.0059†	.0121†	.0203*	-.0020	-.0014
	WI	-.0196	-.0095†	-.0138†	-.0095	.0162	.0030	-.0081	-.0020
7	OUI	-.0051*	-.0028*	-.0059†	.0048†	-.0131*	-.0044*	-.0225**	-.0083
Pearson correlation coefficient between total family income (TFI) and education		.766	.533	.702	.533	.631	.184	.600	.431

*Significant at the 99 percent confidence level.
**Significant at the 95 percent confidence level.
†Significant at the 90 percent confidence level.
NS Less than .00005.

TABLE 30

INCOME COEFFICIENTS, INFANT COHORTS
(EDUCATION EXCLUDED)

	INCOME SPECIFICATION	MALES		FEMALES	
		Blacks	Whites	Blacks	Whites
1	TFI	−.0011	−.0021*	−.0029**	−.0026*
2	UI	.0012	−.0016*	−.0015	−.0024*
	EI	−.0067**	−.0094*	−.0060†	−.0053†
3	UI	−.0007	−.0020*	−.0032**	−.0026*
4	EI	−.0053**	−.0133*	−.0078*	−.0111*
5	TI	−.0035	.0146†	−.0099	.0061
6	SSI	−.0264	.0128	−.0443†	−.0008
	WI	.0066	.0167	.0050	.0142
7	OUI	−.0114	−.0290*	.0091	−.0315*
Pearson correlation coefficient between total family income (TFI) and education[a]		.770	.561	.770	.561

*Significant at the 99 percent confidence level.
**Significant at the 95 percent confidence level.
$\dagger$Significant at the 90 percent confidence level.

a.   Income and education are based on data for women of childbearing age.

These questions were addressed through estimation of a health production function using the mortality rate from all causes as the dependent
variable. The primary empirical extension offered by the work reported
here was estimation of these functions with seven, more refined measures
of income entering the specification. Separate relationships were estimated for 12 population cohorts consisting of three age groups, 0 to 1, 45
to 64, and 65 and older, by sex and race (white and black).

Based on the results reported, the answer to the first question would
seem to be a qualified yes. Analysis of all cohorts and specifications reveals in general a negative relationship. Although a number of the estimated coefficients were statistically insignificant, particularly for adults,
examination of coefficients from variants which excluded education suggested that multicollinearity reduces the reliability of the estimates. At the
same time, however, it is clear that excluding education results in
negatively biased income coefficients.

TABLE 31

Coefficients of Education, All Cohorts[a]

Cohorts	Pearson Correlation Coefficient	Income Included	Income Excluded
Adults			
White males, 45–64	.766	−.0205*	−.0239*
White males, 65+	.533	−.0034	−.0122*
Black males, 45–64	.702	−.0132[†]	−.0203*
Black males, 65+	.533	−.0104[†]	−.0099
White females, 45–64	.631	−.0165**	−.0150*
White females, 65+	.184	−.0203*	−.0233
Black females, 45–64	.600	−.0382*	−.0418*
Black females, 65+	.431	−.0126	−.0099
Male infants			
Whites	.770	−.0522*	−.0754*
Blacks	.561	−.0180	−.0252
Female infants			
Whites	.770	−.0651*	−.0945
Blacks	.560	−.0242	−.0479**

*Significant at the 99 percent confidence level.
**Significant at the 95 percent confidence level.
†Significant at the 90 percent confidence level.

a. Income = total family income (TFI).

With respect to the differential effects of various components of income, our analysis shows that earned income has a negative impact on middle-aged cohorts' mortality rates, but a positive impact on elderly cohorts' mortality rates. The reverse seems to hold true for unearned income. This finding with respect to the effects of earned and unearned income is inconsistent with Silver's study.[8] A plausible explanation of this inconsistency is that Silver's results are probably dominated by results for the elderly, since changes in mortality for these cohorts have a major impact on age-adjusted mortality. However, the results of the pure income transfer variables, WI and OUI, tend to reinforce and clarify Silver's conclusion that higher unearned income contributes to lower mortality rates. Thus, the somewhat ambiguous results for total family income can be better understood when income is broken down into earned and pure transfer components. The impact of the former varies with age, while the latter has a generally negative association with mortality rates for all cohorts.

TABLE 32

INCOME ELASTICITIES, ALL COHORTS

COHORTS	TFI[a]	OUI[a]
Adults		
White males, 45–64	−.071	−.017
White males, 65+	−.020	−.049
Black males, 45–64	−.116	−.005
Black males, 65+	.012	.011
White females, 45–64	−.031	−.039
White females, 65+	.000	−.035
Black females, 45–64	.019	−.013
Black females, 65+	−.011	−.023
Male infants		
Whites	−.187	−.014
Blacks	−.047	−.004
Female infants		
Whites	−.222	−.012
Blacks	−.157	.006

a. Based on coefficients of total family income (TFI) and other unearned income (OUI) from tables 28 and 29, and mean values of TFI and OUI from table 26.

Another indicator of income's effects on mortality is its elasticity, that is, the percentage change in mortality for a small change in income. Table 32 reports elasticities (evaluated at the means) for TFI and OUI, the two variables which most consistently had negative coefficients. These elasticities suggest that income has a negative impact on mortality, but the strength of the relationship is rather weak. For both income variables considered, a 1 percent change in income reduces mortality by about .05 percent on average. The effect is largest for the infant cohorts, with "family income elasticities" ranging from −.047 to −.222. On the other hand, the elasticity of OUI is larger than that for TFI for five of eight adult cohorts.

From a policy viewpoint, these results indicate that income transfer policies aimed at reducing mortality rates will generally contribute to lower mortality, but the magnitude of the effect will not be large. Since reducing mortality rates is not generally the primary motive for income transfers, this conclusion should not be interpreted as a justification for cutting back current income transfer programs. (See chapter 8 for an explicit comparison of an income transfer policy with two alternative policies.)

8

IMPLICATIONS FOR POLICY

The goal of this chapter is to explore the implications of the health production function estimates for several policy issues. Two broad questions underlie this inquiry. How should medical care be allocated across geographic areas and among population cohorts? Is increasing medical care consumption the best policy for reducing mortality rates? Although these questions appear straightforward, answering them requires making explicit assumptions about the criteria used to determine an appropriate allocation of medical care or a best policy for reducing mortality rates. Ultimately, these criteria must be selected by political and social mechanisms that take account of value judgments about the worth of competing outcomes. The purpose of the calculations described in this chapter is to illustrate how the information contained in the health production function can be used to assist in making policy decisions.

The question of medical care resource allocation has several dimensions. Probably the most visible is the distribution of physicians across geographic areas. The principal policy approach to date has been to designate counties, parts of counties, or institutions as health manpower shortage areas or medically underserved areas primarily on the basis of the ratio of population to physicians.[1] Areas with a resident population-per-physician ratio greater than a specified target, currently 3,500 people per nonfederal primary care physician, are designated as underserved.[2] Once designated, the area becomes eligible for a variety of federal programs which place physicians and other health personnel in underserved areas.

The main advantage of this approach is its simplicity. However, use of the population-to-physician ratio has several well-known shortcomings: the choice of the cutoff point, 3,500 to 1, is arbitrary; a single-valued

113

threshold takes no account of gradations in the degree of underservice; and focusing on the stock of available physicians ignores differences in the demand for medical care, the actual use of services, the health levels of the population, the use of other nonphysician resources, and the impact of additional physicians on health. Finally, the population-to-physician ratio may have an inherent bias in favor of rural areas because it ignores travel patterns to obtain care and because of the difficulty of identifying intra-county shortages, especially in large urban areas. As will be illustrated, criteria developed from the health production function take some of these factors into account.

Another aspect of the distribution issue is the allocation of medical care among population groups. The Medicare and Medicaid programs, for example, have increased medical care use by the elderly, the poor, and other persons eligible for coverage. The Carter administration's CHAP (Children's Health Assessment Program) legislation, if it had been enacted, would probably have had a similar impact on the use of medical care by children. These programs are based primarily on observations of differences in the use of medical care by various population groups and presumptions about the likely benefits of more medical care consumption. The age-sex-race-specific health production functions estimated may provide more precise information for making decisions on these programs.

The comparison between increasing medical care use and other policies for reducing mortality rates have received little explicit analysis. Several studies have questioned whether additional medical care would contribute anything at all to the goal of reducing mortality rates.[3] In effect, these studies argue that medical care's marginal product in the health production function is zero. Other analyses have claimed that mortality rates are primarily a function of environmental and behavior factors, and that medical care's impact is relatively insignificant, though not necessarily zero.[4] It follows, then, that policy should be directed at changing the environment or behavior rather than increasing medical care consumption.

The results reported in chapters 5 and 6 show clearly that the marginal product of medical care is not zero. The validity of the second contention, that increasing medical care use is an inefficient policy, is much more difficult to access. The main problem is that little is known about the costs of changing the environment or changing behavior. Unless information about the costs of alternative policies is also considered, choices among policy options will be based on incomplete data. Thus, a third goal of this chapter is to make exploratory comparisons among the policies of increasing medical care use, increasing family income, and reducing cigarette consumption. This phase of the analysis is again meant to be illustrative, since the data are crude and only three alternative policies will be examined.

Policy Goals and Evaluation Criteria

Improving health is clearly one of the primary goals underlying each of these policy questions. In and of itself, however, the simply stated goal "improving health" has two major flaws as a criterion for evaluating alternative policies. The first is that it has no operational content. It is too general and too vague to be useful. As discussed in chapter 4, defining and measuring health are extremely difficult. The second flaw is that "improving health" is an unbounded and unconstrained goal. How much should health be improved? Is any improvement in health, no matter how small, an acceptable criterion? What are the limits on the resources which can be used to improve health?

The first of these two problems is dealt with by using the mortality rate as an inverse health indicator. In effect, it is assumed that the general goal of improving health can be represented by the more specific and more easily measurable objective of lowering mortality rates. The second problem, bounding the amount of health improvement, is approached in two ways. One assumes that the policy goal is to achieve the greatest health improvement (mortality reduction) possible for a given budget or resource expenditure. The other poses the policy goal as reaching a well-defined health improvement target, that is, a predetermined decrease in mortality rates. Implicitly, the second approach permits the policy to use whatever resources necessary to reach the desired target.

The health production functions developed and estimated in preceding chapters provide both the conceptual and empirical foundations for identifying and comparing alternative policies. Medical care use, behavioral factors, and environmental conditions are inputs into the health production function. Policies to reduce mortality rates are in essence policies to alter the levels or values of health production function inputs. Efforts to increase medical care use, reduce cigarette consumption, increase income, and improve air quality are straightforward examples of trying to change health production function inputs. This framework also clearly illustrates the distinction between an intermediate goal, for example, increasing medical care use, and the ultimate goal of reducing mortality rates.

Given the conceptual framework, the production function's parameters provide the means of deriving numerical estimates of each policy's impact on mortality rates. In particular, for any geographic area and population cohort, the change in the mortality rate can be defined as

$$\Delta Y_{ij} = \zeta_j Y_{ij}(\Delta X_{ij}/X_{ij}), \tag{8.1}$$

where

ΔY_{ij} = the change in the mortality rate in the ith geographic area for the jth population cohort,

Y_{ij} = the existing mortality rate,

$(\Delta X_{ij}/X_{ij})$ = the percentage change in the value of input X in the ith geographic area for the jth population cohort, and

ζ_j = the elasticity of the mortality rate with respect to input X.

The elasticity, which is simply the percentage change in the mortality rate associated with a small, typically 1 percent, change in the value of an input, can be computed directly from the estimated values of the health production function's parameters.[5] (Note that in this formulation the parameter values, and thus the elasticity estimates, vary across cohorts but not across individual geographic areas.) The advantages of using equation (8.1) to measure a policy's impact on mortality rates are twofold. First, the elasticity estimates, ζ_j, are direct measures of each input's contribution to health production when other factors are held constant. Inputs which have a large impact on mortality rates will have large elasticities. Second, the area-cohort-specific change in the mortality rate depends on existing values of both the mortality rate, Y_{ij}, and the policy variable (input), X_{ij}.

One can think of ΔY_{ij} as the benefit or payoff from changing one of the production function's inputs. This benefit can be aggregated to the area or cohort level simply by summing over cohorts or geographic areas, respectively. However, knowing a policy's payoff is only one of the essential ingredients needed to compare alternative policies. Another is the cost of the policy. (Others, such as political feasibility, distributional consequences, and administrative feasibility will not be considered here.) Therefore, the general evaluation criterion which will be used in the following policy simulations is the number of deaths averted per $100,000 of policy cost. (The inverse of this indicator is the cost of lowering the relevant mortality rate by one death per year.) For example, the policy of increasing medical care use will be assessed using the number of deaths averted per $100,000 increase in medical care spending, which will be referred to as DAMC, as an evaluation criterion. The advantage of this criterion is that it incorporates both the policy's impact on mortality rates (deaths averted) and the policy's costs. Furthermore, since the estimate of the number of deaths averted is derived from the health production function, the criterion implicitly takes into account health levels in the local area, the current value of the policy variable (medical care use) in the local area, and medical care's importance in health production (through its elasticity with respect to the mortality rate).

Given the evaluation criterion, one still needs to know how the policy is to be constrained. Consider the following example. Suppose that the government has decided to increase spending for medical care by a certain amount and wants to know the best allocation of the additional funds across counties. Suppose further that equity considerations limit the amount by which spending can be increased in any particular county.[6] For example, one can imagine a policy which grants each county resident a voucher worth ΔMC dollars of increased medical care consumption if the county qualifies for the grant, and no voucher otherwise. (One can also interpret a program like the National Health Services Corp (NHSC), which places federally supported physicians in medical practices as a conceptually similar policy, since the NHSC is effectively a subsidy for medical care use in the practice's location.) The questions, then, are which counties should receive the grant and in what order?

The answers to these questions clearly depend on how the policy is constrained. One plausible approach is to limit the amount of money available and to maximize the total number of deaths averted for the given increase in expenditures. It then follows that counties should be ranked in descending order on the basis of the value of DAMC, the number of deaths averted per $100,000 increase in medical care spending. Starting with the county with the largest value of DAMC and making grants until the policy's budget is exhausted will maximize the number of deaths averted.

The alternative approach to bounding the policy fixes the amount of health improvement to be attained. For example, this is one way to view the question of how many additional physicians are "needed" in a county. Need, of course, has to be defined relative to some objective. In particular, assume that the policy objective is to reduce age-sex-race-specific mortality rates to the level of the national average for each cohort in 1970. Thus, define the target decrease in the mortality rate, ΔY^*_{ij}, as

$$\Delta Y^*_{ij} = \begin{cases} \overline{Y}_j - Y_{ij} \text{ if } Y_{ij} > \overline{Y}_j \\ \\ 0 \text{ if } Y_{ij} \leq \overline{Y}_j \end{cases} \tag{8.2}$$

where $\overline{Y}_j$ is the cohort-specific national average mortality rate. Equation (8.2) states that the target decrease in the mortality rate is zero if the cohort's actual mortality rate in the county, Y_{ij}, is less than or equal to the national average mortality rate for that cohort, $\overline{Y}_j$. If Y_{ij} exceeds $\overline{Y}_j$, then the target decrease is equal to the difference $\overline{Y}_j - Y_{ij}$. Given the values of the targets for each county and cohort, one can rewrite equation (8.1) to solve for ΔMC^*_{ij}, the needed change in medical care expenditures per capita:

$$\Delta MC^*_{ij} = \frac{\Delta Y^*_{ij}}{Y_{ij}} \cdot \frac{MC_{ij}}{\zeta_j} \geq 0 \qquad (8.2)$$

In order to translate this into needed physicians, it is necessary to estimate the relationship between medical expenditures and the supply of physicians.[7]

The solution to this problem assumes that no resources are reallocated from one location to another, since ΔY_{ij} is set to zero if Y_{ij} is less than the national average. If the policy goal were to equalize cohort-specific mortality rates across counties, than ΔY^*_{ij} would be permitted to have positive values, implying that some areas would lose medical care resources. Clearly, the total additional medical care resources required would be less than if only net increases in expenditures were to occur.

Neither of these two examples is particularly realistic in the sense that it accurately reflects current policy options. Nevertheless, the key variables computed may be very useful as indices for ranking counties in terms of their need for additional medical care. Two questions are of particular interest for policy purposes. First, how closely related is a ranking based on DAMC or ΔMC^* with a ranking based on the population-to-physician ratio? If the correlations are high, then the current method of designating shortage areas would be reinforced. If the correlations are not high, then the related question is, what other readily available county data are highly correlated with the ranking criteria developed from the health production function?

On *a priori* grounds, the DAMC criterion seems to have several advantages compared to the population-to-physician ratio. First, DAMC takes account of current health levels through the values of Y_{ij} (current mortality rates), the efficiency of health production through ζ_j, and current medical care consumption levels, X_{ij}. (The deaths-averted criterion weights all lives equally. An alternative but related criterion is the years-of-life-saved per \$100,000 increase in medical spending. This criterion would clearly weight an infant's death averted more heavily than a retired person's death averted.)

Second, DAMC is neutral with respect to an area's population size. The population-to-physician ratio has a clear bias toward less populated areas because this measure is able to correct only very imperfectly for people's travel patterns to obtain medical care. DAMC avoids this problem by measuring both medical care consumption and mortality rates by place of residence rather than place of occurrence.

Third, cardinal comparisons of DAMC across counties have a clear interpretation. A county with a value of DAMC twice as large as that of another county would have twice as many deaths averted for equal expenditure increases in each county. Conversely, if the goal were to attain equal reductions in mortality rates, it would require twice as large an increase in expenditures in the county with the lower value of DAMC.

A second dimension of the medical care resource allocation issue concerns the allocation among population groups. The estimates of the cohort-specific health production functions can also be applied to this question by computing cohort-specific estimates of the number of deaths averted per dollar increase in medical care spending, $DAMC_j$. This estimate could be averaged over counties (or, alternatively, be computed with national data) in order to obtain aggregate estimates of whether there are significant differences among population groups in the expected payoff from consuming more medical care. Although there is little precedent or likelihood of developing subsidy programs which are sex-and/or race-specific, there is ample precedent for age-specific subsidies, for example, Medicare. Of particular interest is the comparison between the infant cohorts and the two adult cohorts. If the former are more responsive (have a larger value of DAMC), then this would strengthen the case for developing a program such as CHAP.

The final area of policy application is the comparison among different approaches to reducing mortality rates. Again, the basis for comparison will be the number of lives saved per dollar spent under a particular policy. Increasing family incomes by 10 percent and reducing cigarette consumption by 10 percent are the two policies which will be compared to increased medical care use. Estimates of the elasticities of the mortality rate with respect to family income and cigarette consumption will be derived from the health production functions estimated in chapters 5 and 6. Summing the numbers of deaths averted over cohorts and geographic areas (or using national data) would produce national estimates of the number of deaths averted. Dividing these estimates by the cost of each policy provides a basis for evaluating the relative efficiency of expanding medical care consumption, reducing cigarette consumption, and increasing family incomes as policies for reducing mortality rates.

These policy simulations have been described in general terms without specific reference to the data used to estimate the health production function. Several additional assumptions must be made explicit, however, before the results of the simulations are reported. First, it is assumed that the estimated functions represent the long-run relationship between mortality rates and the other variables. Thus, the contemplated policy changes should be thought of as permanent, one-time shifts which result in movement to a new equilibrium on the health production function. (For example, in terms of figure 2 in chapter 2, an increase in medical care spending is interpreted as a shift of the supply function for medical care in quadrant 3.)

Second, the parameters of the health production function are assumed to be independent of the geographic unit of analysis. Thus, the parameters estimated with data for county groups will be applied to both county and national data. Focusing on the county in the policy simulations is of particular relevance since this is the geographic unit most frequently used in designating medical shortage areas.

Third, the ratio of Medicare expenditures per enrollee is assumed to be a constant fraction (across areas) of the various age-sex-race-specific measures of medical expenditures per capita. These ratios will be computed from national data on per capita medical care expenditures by cohort.

The lack of sufficiently detailed data on medical care spending and other population characteristics at the local level is the primary reason for making these assumptions. Although they appear to be strong assumptions, they are really much less restrictive than the implicit assumptions underlying, for example, the use of the population-to-physician ratio as a criterion for designating shortage areas. Furthermore, making these assumptions explicit clearly indicates the types of information which would be needed to relax them.

Policy Simulations

This section reports the methods and results of the policy simulations. The estimation of cohort-specific medical care spending is described first. This is followed by the computations of $DAMC_i$, the number of deaths averted per dollar increase in medical care spending across counties. We then address the question of how closely DAMC is correlated both with the population-to-physician ratio and with other data available at the county level. Cohort-specific estimates, $DAMC_j$, are reported next. The fourth issue investigated is the need for additional physicians. Finally increased medical care spending is compared with two alternative policies: reducing cigarette consumption per capita and increasing family incomes.

One additional problem which arises with the use of county data is the instability of annual death rates in counties with small populations.[8] Since the mortality rate is an integral component of the calculations reported, there is a tendency for small counties to take on extreme values in some cases. In order to test the sensitivity of the results to the presence of outliers, findings are reported both for all counties and for counties with at least 2,000 people in the cohorts analyzed. This eliminates about 10 percent of all counties (360) from consideration.

1. COHORT-SPECIFIC ESTIMATES OF MEDICAL CARE EXPENDITURES

Estimation of the health production function for each cohort required the assumption that cohort-specific medical care expenditures per capita are a constant proportion (across areas) of Medicare expenditures per enrollee. It was not necessary, however, to know the numerical value of that proportion. Several of the policy simulations, on the other hand, do require estimates of cohort-specific spending for medical care.

National data on age-sex-race-specific expenditures for medical care in 1970 do not exist. Estimates of per capita expenditures by age, sex, or race are available from a survey of more than 10,000 households, conducted by the Center for Health Administration Studies and the National Opinion Research Corporation (CHAS-NORC). This survey was designed to be representative of the entire U.S. population.[9] Data on medical expenditures for three age groups are reported by the Social Security Administration (SSA).[10]

Table 33 summarizes this information. Data from the CHAS-NORC survey are similar to the SSA data for each age group except those 65 and older, where the SSA estimate is 43 percent larger. The probable explanation for this is that the CHAS-NORC household survey excluded institutionalized people and those potential respondents who lived alone and died during the survey period.[11] The estimates for all ages are nearly identical, however, since the population excluded by CHAS-NORC is a very small proportion of the total population. As expected, expenditures per capita generally increase with age. (The slightly higher expenditures in the CHAS-NORC data for ages 18–34 compared to ages 35–54 probably reflects childbearing expenses for younger women.)

Differences in spending by race are relatively large, with blacks consuming only about two-thirds as much medical care as whites. Since the CHAS-NORC estimates include the value of free care (Medicaid, welfare,

TABLE 33
ESTIMATES OF PER CAPITA MEDICAL CARE EXPENDITURES
BY AGE, RACE, AND SEX, 1970

	CHAS-NORC[a] ($)	SSA[b] ($)
Age groups		
0–5	110	
6–17	112	113[c]
18–34	283	
35–54	249	273[d]
55–64	378	
65+	438	625
All ages	248	249
Race		
White	259	
		NA
Nonwhite	173	
Sex		
Male	237	
		NA
Female	260	
Medicare expenditures per enrollee–$325		

SOURCES: CHAS-NORC—U.S. Department of Health, Education and Welfare, Health
Resources Administration, *Expenditures for Personal Health Services: National Trends and Variations 1953–1970.* p. 45; HEW, Social Security Administration (SSA), *Compendium of National Health Expenditures Data,* p. 81; Medicare, HEW, SSA, *Medicare 1970,* p. 9.
  a. Includes spending for hospitals, physicians, drugs, dental services, and other health practitioners.
  b. Includes spending for hospitals, physicians, dentists, drugs, and other professional services.
  c. 0–19 years old.
  d. 20–64 years old.
NA Not available.

local governments, and other entitlement programs such as V.A.), the difference probably reflects real differences in consumption. Differences in consumption by sex are slight, however, with spending by males 91 percent of that for females.

Although the CHAS-NORC data appear to be reliable overall, we shall use the SSA estimate of spending for the elderly, since the mortality data for this study include the entire population in each cohort and not just the noninstitutionalized population. The estimate of spending for infants' medical care and for the 45 to 64 age group will be taken from the CHAS-NORC data. The former is $110 and the latter will be assumed to be $314, the average of the spending levels reported for the 35 to 54 and 55 to 64 age groups. Within each age group, we assume that blacks spend two-thirds as much as whites. However, differences in spending by sex are ignored. Finally, the analysis of infant mortality (chapter 6) implicitly assumed that medical care spending during pregnancy and birth is integral to explaining infant mortality rates. Therefore, an estimate of total medical care spending per live birth, also from the CHAS-NORC survey, of $646 will be added to the $110 estimates of medical care spending for infants.[12]

Following the basic assumption of the production function estimation, the ratio of age-race-specific medical care expenditures per capita to the national average Medicare expenditures per enrollee was computed. These proportionality constants were then applied to the county-specific data on Medicare expenditures per enrollee in order to generate cohort-specific estimates of per capita and total medical care spending in each county. (The latter was computed by multiplying each per capita estimate by the population of the relevant cohort.)

The resulting proportionality constants for whites are 2.30 for infants, 0.97 for 45 to 64 years olds, and 1.92 for those 65 and older. Thus, for example, the estimate of total medical care spending for prenatal, obstetrical, and infant health care per white infant in each county is obtained by multiplying each county's reported data on Medicare expenditures per enrollee residing in the county by 2.30. Estimates of per capita spending for all medical care services in the other two cohorts are obtained in the same way. Estimates for black cohorts are assumed to be 66 percent those for whites.

2. DEATHS AVERTED BY INCREASED MEDICAL CARE SPENDING AND MEDICAL CARE RESOURCE ALLOCATION

Applying the proportionality constants to county data on Medicare expenditures per enrollee produces an estimate of $359 per capita for medical care spending by people in the 12 cohorts in the analysis. This implies that these cohort members spent a total of just over $23 billion for personal health services in 1970, which was about 50 percent of total U.S. medical spending. The cohorts' high per capita spending level and their disproportionate share of total medical spending (these cohorts comprised approximately 35 percent of the entire population) are the result of high expenditures associated with old age, childbirth, and infant care. If the policy under consideration is to increase medical care spending by 10 percent for these cohorts, then the total cost of this policy would be about $2.3 billion.

The number of deaths averted by this policy is computed directly from equation (8.1). This calculation results in an estimate of 27,827 deaths averted over all cohorts. The mortality rate of 27.99 deaths per 1,000 people is reduced by 1.61 percent. Combining the estimates of the benefits and costs of the policy results in a national average of 1.21 deaths averted per $100,000 increase in medical care spending for these cohorts.

At the county level the number of deaths averted per $100,000 increase in medical care spending ranges from a minimum of 0.2 to a maximum of 3.8. It is higher the larger the cohort-specific mortality rates and the greater the presence of high mortality cohorts in the county. Excluding counties with fewer than 2,000 people or 50 deaths had only a minimal impact on the calculations—the mean value of DAMC increased to 1.4, but the standard deviation, minimum, and maximum values of the distribution were unchanged.

What is the correlation between DAMC and other criteria used to designate medically underserved areas? As noted, the principal criterion currently used is the number of people per active, nonfederal primary care physician in the county. Other possible criteria are the number of people per active, nonfederal, patient care physician, the mortality rate, Medicare expenditures per enrollee, and an indicator of medical care use relative to the need for care (the ratio of Medicare expenditures per enrollee to the mortality rate). Data limitations require that primary care physicians be defined as general practitioners, medical specialists, and osteopaths. This incorrectly includes medical and pediatric subspecialists and excludes obstetrician-gynecologists and general surgeons who provide primary care. The distortion should not be large, however. Also, the mortality rate used in the correlations reported applies only to the cohorts used in this study.[13]

Table 34 reports the Pearson correlation coefficients among the potential allocation criteria.[14] DAMC has positive correlations with both population per primary care physician (POPPC) and population per patient care physician (POPMD), that is, counties with large values of the number of deaths averted per $100,000 increase in medical care spending also tend to have large populations relative to the numbers of physicians in the county. However, the magnitudes of the correlations are relatively low, only 0.18 and 0.22 respectively.

TABLE 34
CORRELATIONS BETWEEN DEATHS AVERTED PER $100,000 INCREASE IN MEDICAL
CARE SPENDING AND OTHER ALLOCATION CRITERIA ($n = 3068$)

	DAMC	POPPC	POPMD	MR	MDCREXP	USENEED
DAMC	1.00					
POPPC	0.18	1.00				
POPMD	0.22	0.83	1.00			
MR	0.47	−0.08	0.01	1.00		
MDCREXP	−0.83	−0.18	−0.21	−0.18	1.00	
USENEED	−0.82	−0.09	−0.15	−0.60	0.85	1.00

Key: DAMC   — Deaths averted per $100,000 increase in medical care spending.
POPPC   — Population per active, nonfederal primary care physician.
POPMD   — Population per active, nonfederal patient care physician.
MR   — Deaths per 1,000 people (study cohorts only).
MDCREXP — Medicare expenditures per enrollee.
USENEED — Ratio of MDCREXP to MR.

It is possible that DAMC and the two population-per-physician ratios are more highly correlated when one examines only counties with the largest values in the tails of the respective ranking criteria. Accordingly, counties were ranked both by POPMD and by DAMC, and the Pearson correlation coefficients were recomputed for the 500 counties with the largest values of POPMD and DAMC, respectively. (The POPMD ranking included counties with no physicians.) In both cases, the correlations remained very low.[15] In addition, only 111 counties appear in the upper tails of both distributions. Thus, the weak relationship between DAMC and population-per-physician ratios holds even for counties with the largest values in each distribution.

DAMC has a moderately high correlation of 0.47 with the mortality rate, MR. However, the largest correlations are with Medicare expenditures per enrollee, MDCREXP, and the use-need ratio (USENEED—the ratio of MDCREXP to MR). The correlation coefficients are about −0.80. The former is assumed to be a proxy for medical care consumption by the county's residents and the latter a measure of medical care consumption relative to health. The negative correlation between DAMC and these two variables means that counties which have large values of DAMC tend to be relatively low consumers of medical care, both absolutely and relative to need (as approximated by the mortality rate). When only the 500 counties with the largest values of DAMC are considered, the correlation between DAMC and MDCREXP is smaller in absolute value, -0.59. However, the correlation with USENEED remains virtually unchanged, -0.81.

The high correlation between DAMC and USENEED should not be surprising, since the two are in fact functionally related. This can be readily seen by rewriting equation (8.1) as

$$\frac{\Delta Y_{ij}}{\Delta MC_{ij}} = \zeta_j \frac{Y_{ij}}{MC_{ij}} \tag{8.3}$$

The left-hand side of (8.3) is the general definition of the change in the mortality rate for a given change in medical care expenditures per capita. DAMC is simply the value of this ratio normalized for a particular increase in medical care spending, \$100,000. The ratio Y_{ij}/MC_{ij} is a variant of USENEED, the ratio of cohort- and county-specific mortality rates to medical care spending per capita. Finally, the ζ_j are the cohort-specific coefficient estimates from the health production function. Since $\zeta_j < 0$ and given the simple relationship expressed by (8.3), DAMC and USENEED will have a large, negative correlation.

Finally, it is quite interesting to note the low correlations among POPPC and POPMD, and the three proxies for need for and use of services, MR, MDCREXP, and USENEED. Together, these correlations suggest that there is little relationship between the *availability* of physicians in a county and its residents' use of medical care services or their health status (as approximated by the mortality rate). One explanation of this result is that county borders bear little relation to medical care market areas. Market area size depends on patients' travel patterns and the geographic concentrations of physicians in different medical specialties. (Clearly, specialists are likely to have larger trade areas than generalists.) Consequently, POPPC and POPMD are poor indicators of medical underservice or the need for more medical care. Overall, if it is agreed that DAMC is an acceptable allocation criterion, then the ratio of Medicare expenditures per enrollee to the mortality rate appears to be a highly correlated and readily available proxy criterion.

As was noted, only 111 counties were included in both sets of the 500 counties with the largest values of DAMC and POPMD. Other differences in the geographic distributions of these counties are shown in table 35 and maps 1-4. Diagonal lines indicate counties with large values of POPMD;

TABLE 35
PERCENTAGE DISTRIBUTION OF MEDICALLY NEEDY COUNTIES BY
CENSUS DIVISION AND REGION FOR TWO RANKING CRITERIA

| | CRITERION | |
	POPULATION PER PHYSICIAN (POPMD) (n = 500) %	DEATHS AVERTED PER $100,000 INCREASE IN MEDICAL CARE SPENDING (DAMC) (n = 500) %
Census Division		
New England	0.2	0.4
Mid-Atlantic	0.2	2.2
South Atlantic	21.6	41.4
East South Central	14.2	26.4
West South Central	17.0	14.6
East North Central	8.2	6.2
West North Central	28.2	6.2
Mountain	8.2	2.6
Pacific	2.2	0.0
Census Region		
Northeast	0.4	2.6
South	52.8	82.4
North Central	36.4	12.4
West	10.4	2.6

dots denote counties with large values of DAMC; and counties which are members of both sets are shown by the overlap of diagonal lines and dots.) Neither criterion includes many counties in either the northeast (map 1) or western (map 4) regions. However, there are fairly dramatic differences between the two in both the southern (map 2) and north central (map 3) regions. The POPMD criterion places 36.4 percent of its 500 counties in the north central region. By contrast, the DAMC criterion includes only 12.4 percent of its counties in this region, but 82.4 percent in the southern region. The main reason for this shift is that while it is true that many north central (and western) counties are geographically remote and have

MAP 1

COUNTIES WITH LARGE VALUES OF TWO RANKING CRITERIA,
NORTHEASTERN, NORTH CENTRAL, AND MIDDLE ATLANTIC STATES, 1970

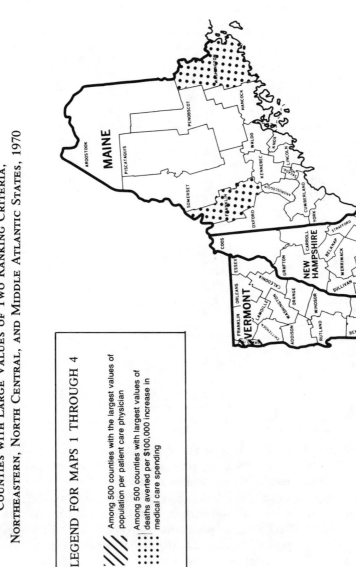

LEGEND FOR MAPS 1 THROUGH 4

Among 500 counties with the largest values of
population per patient care physician

Among 500 counties with largest values of
deaths averted per $100,000 increase in
medical care spending

© RAND McNALLY & COMPANY, R. L. 81-Y-21

MAP 1 (cont'd)

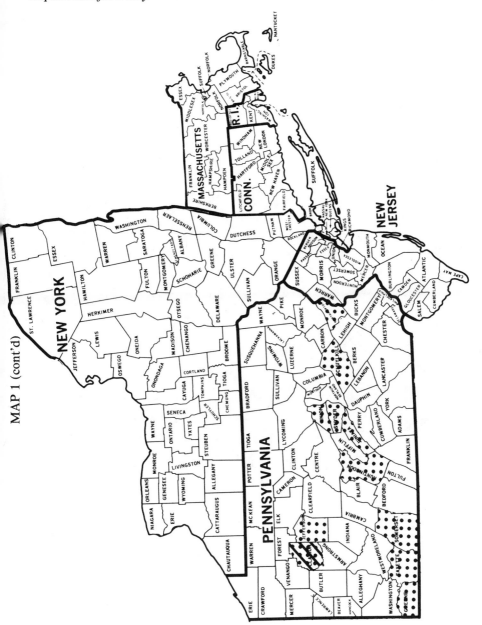

MAP 1 (cont'd)

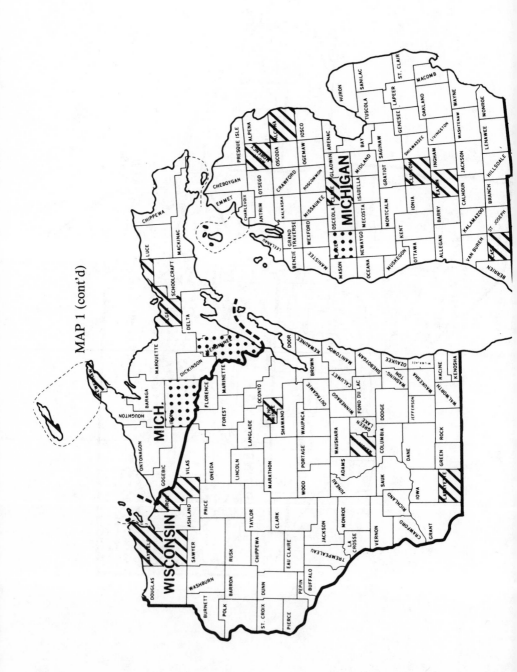

MAP 1 (cont'd)

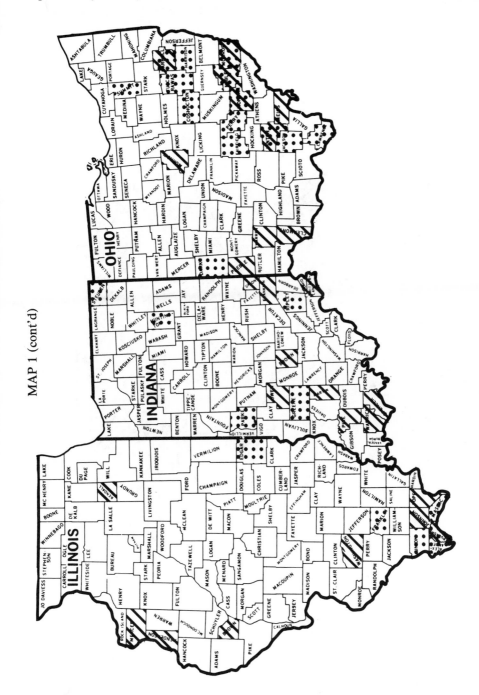

MAP 2

Counties with Large Values of Two Ranking Criteria, South Atlantic and East South Central States, 1970

See legend on page 128.

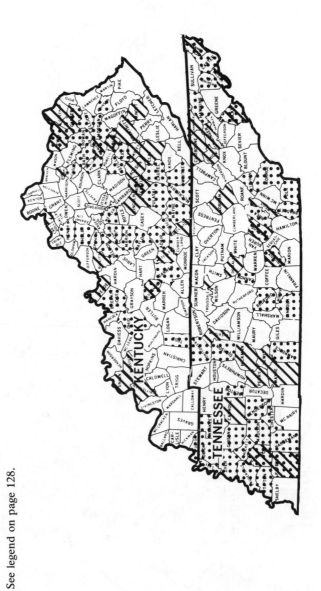

© RAND McNALLY & COMPANY, R. L. 81-Y-21

MAP 2 (cont'd)

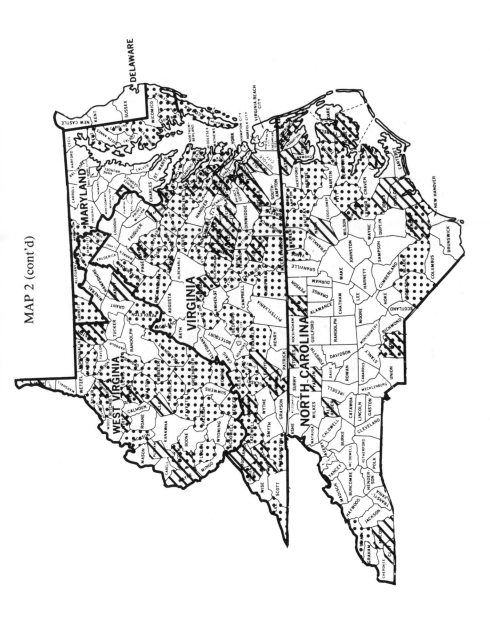

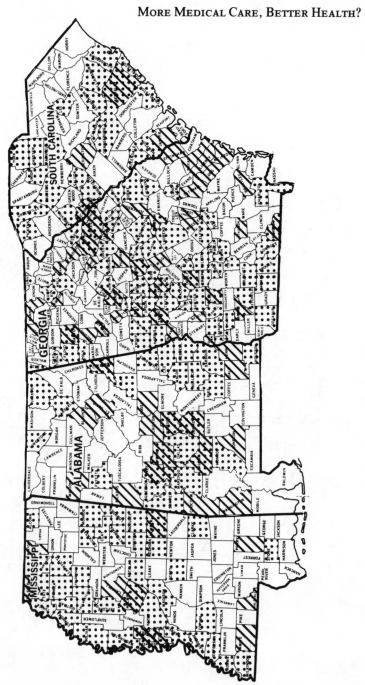

MAP 2 (cont'd)

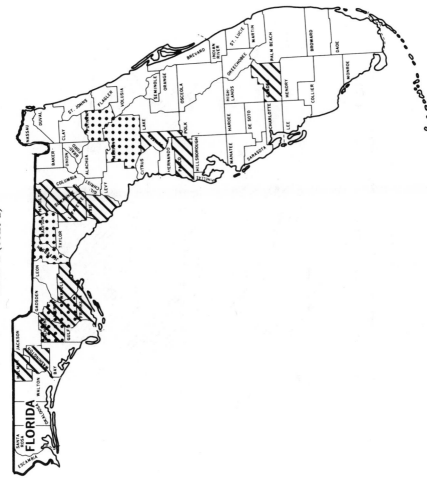

MAP 2 (cont'd)

MAP 3
COUNTIES WITH LARGE VALUES OF TWO RANKING CRITERIA, WEST
NORTH CENTRAL AND WEST SOUTH CENTRAL STATES, 1970

See legend on page 128.

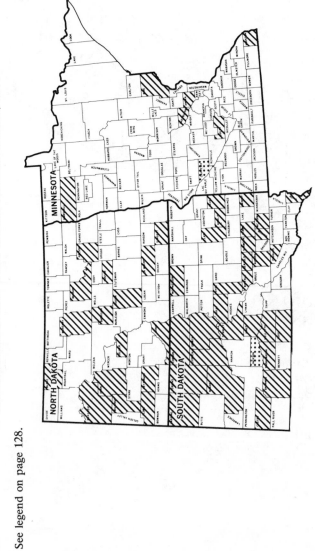

MAP 3 (cont'd)

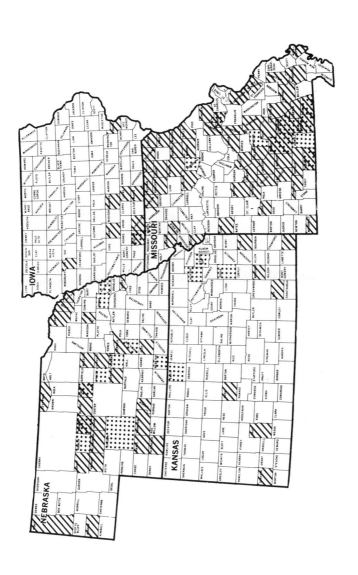

MAP 3 (cont'd)

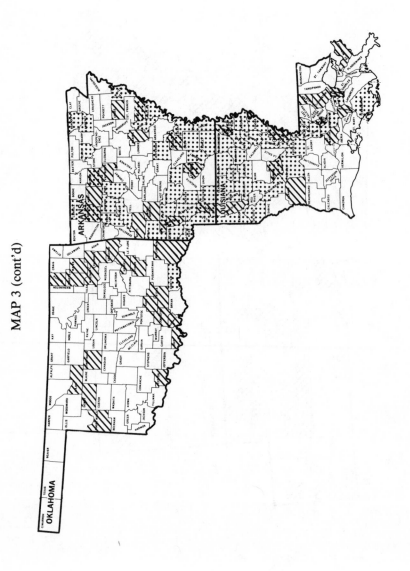

MAP 3 (cont'd)

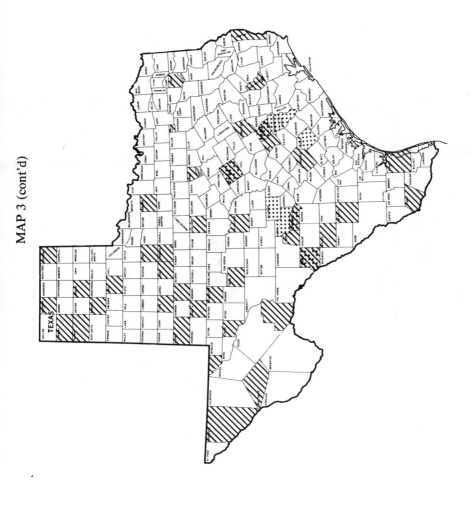

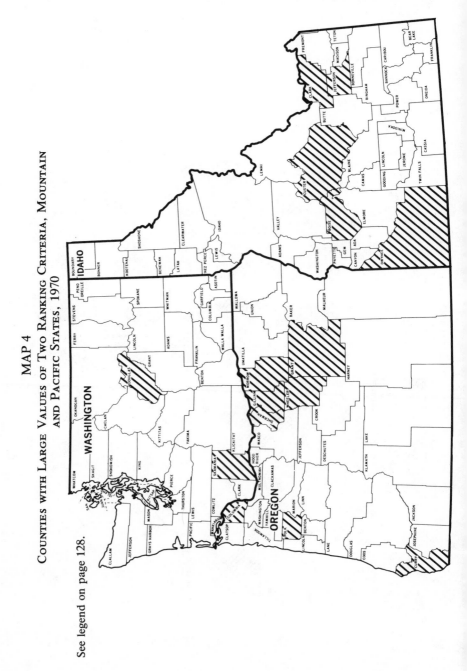

MAP 4

Counties with Large Values of Two Ranking Criteria, Mountain and Pacific States, 1970

See legend on page 128.

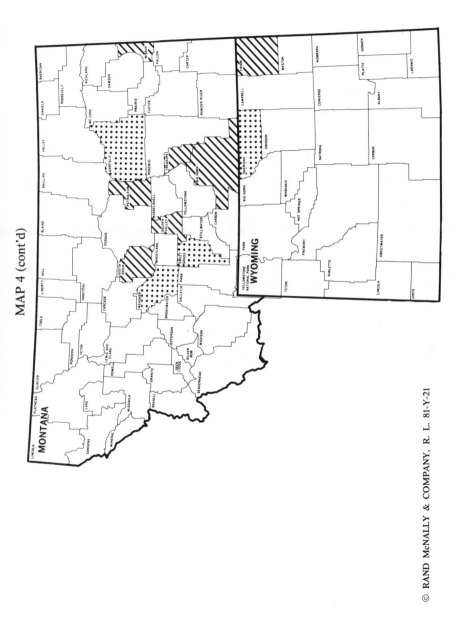

MAP 4 (cont'd)

© RAND McNALLY & COMPANY, R. L. 81-Y-21

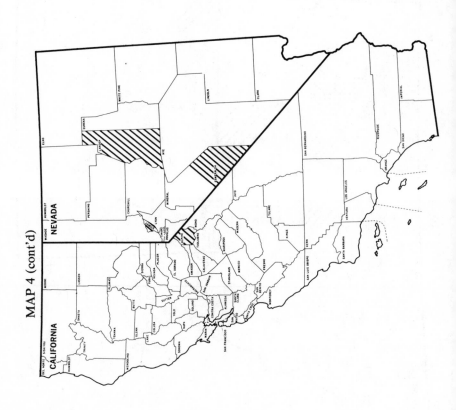

MAP 4 (cont'd)

MAP 4 (cont'd)

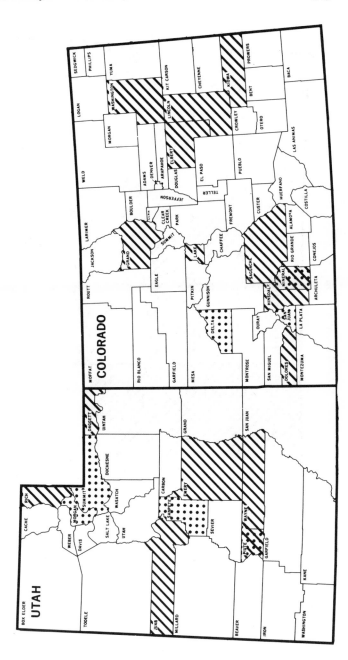

MAP 4 (cont'd)

few physicians, their populations appear to have better underlying health status. Thus, one of the main effects of using DAMC rather than POPMD as an allocation criterion would be to shift a greater share of additional resources to the southern region. (Appendix B provides larger scale and more detailed maps for selected states.)

In terms of the distribution of these counties by population size groups, both criteria tend to concentrate on counties in the smaller size categories. Table 36 shows the distributions across the American Medical Association's county population size classifications. As can be seen, the main difference is in the number of counties which are in the smallest size category. More than 50 percent of the counties in the POPMD ranking are

TABLE 36
DISTRIBUTION OF MEDICALLY NEEDY COUNTIES BY POPULATION SIZE GROUP,
FOR TWO RANKING CRITERIA

	CRITERION	
	POPULATION PER PHYSICIAN (POPMD) (n = 500) %	DEATHS AVERTED PER $100,000 INCREASE IN MEDICAL CARE SPENDING (DAMC) (n = 500) %
County Population Size[a]		
Nonmetro., 0-9,999 inhabitants	55.4	22.4
Nonmetro., 10,000-24,999 inhabitants	26.4	43.5
Nonmetro., 25,000-49,999 inhabitants	4.0	18.0
Nonmetro., 50,000+ inhabitants	0.8	7.0
Potential SMSAs	0.4	0.2
Metro, 50,000-499,999 inhabitants	7.2	6.6
Metro, 500,000-999,999 inhabitants	2.8	1.8
Metro, 1,000,000-4,999,999 inhabitants	3.0	0.6
Metro, 5,000,000+ inhabitants	0.0	0.0

a. American Medical Association definitions.

nonmetropolitan with fewer than 10,000 inhabitants, compared to just over 20 percent of the counties ranked by DAMC. In both cases, however, more than 85 percent of the counties are nonmetropolitan.

Neither criterion appears well suited for identifying medically needy areas at the subcounty level. This is a potentially severe problem for the most populous metropolitan counties. Many of these are thought to have large population pockets which receive inadequate medical care. In principle, DAMC can be computed for any size geographic area if data on medical care expenditures and mortality rates are available by age, sex, and race. Such data are generally not available, however. Thus, identifying subcounty medical care shortage areas will probably continue to be an interactive process involving both aggregate criteria, such as POPMD or DAMC, and locally supplied information.

3. MEDICAL CARE RESOURCE ALLOCATION ACROSS POPULATION GROUPS

This section reports calculations of the numbers of deaths averted per $100,000 increase in medical care spending for each of the cohorts for which a health production function was estimated. Two policy questions underlie these calculations. Are there significant differences in DAMC by age group? Are there significant differences by race? The former has implications for programs such as Medicare and CHAP (The Child Health Assessment Program), while the latter is relevant to the development of programs aimed at improving minorities' health. Since many counties have very small populations in some age-sex-race categories (particularly for blacks), calculations are reported both for all counties and for counties with at least 10 deaths in a cohort. In general, observed mortality rates will be more reliable indicators of underlying health status in the latter counties.

Table 37 reports the calculations of DAMC for each cohort. Several patterns emerge from these data. First, with the exception of white males, the elderly cohorts have the largest values of DAMC for each sex-race combination. Second, except for middle-age males, black cohorts have larger values of DAMC than white cohorts within each sex-age group. Further, these racial differences are fairly large, with values of DAMC usually two to three times greater for blacks than for whites. Third, differences by sex are relatively small, except for middle-aged whites. Finally, limiting the calculations to counties with at least 10 deaths in a cohort has little impact on the mean values of DAMC, although it significantly reduces the standard deviations (and numbers of counties). Thus,

TABLE 37
DEATHS AVERTED PER $100,000 INCREASE
IN MEDICAL CARE SPENDING BY COHORT

COHORT	ALL COUNTIES			COUNTIES WITH AT LEAST TEN DEATHS IN COHORT		
	Mean	S.D.	n	Mean	S.D.	n
White males, 45–64	1.9	0.6	3,068	2.0	0.6	2,548
White males, 65+	1.8	0.5	3,068	1.8	0.5	2,929
Black males, 45–64	1.1	1.4	2,413	1.2	0.4	595
Black males, 65+	3.9	3.4	2,281	3.8	1.2	815
White females, 45–64	0.3	0.1	3,068	0.3	0.1	1,753
White females, 65+	1.4	0.4	3,068	1.4	0.4	2,874
Black females, 45–64	1.3	2.0	2,413	1.5	0.5	455
Black females, 65+	3.0	3.1	2,300	2.9	0.9	747
White male infants	0.5	0.5	3,072	0.5	0.2	680
Black male infants	1.3	2.5	1,838	1.4	0.7	202
White female infants	0.4	0.5	3,074	0.4	0.2	499
Black female infants	1.3	2.6	1,824	1.4	0.8	157

inferences based on the larger number of counties seem warranted, even with the large standard deviations associated with the black cohorts.

These results would seem to support programs aimed at increasing medical care use by the elderly and by racial minorities. However, they do not show a clearcut advantage for programs targeted at increasing medical care consumption for pregnancy, childbirth, and infants, at least for whites. This last inference needs to be qualified in two ways. First, the underlying calculations assume that all spending associated with childbirth should be allocated to infant health. If in fact some share of that spending should be attributed to maternal health, then the value of DAMC will be proportionately larger. (If all childbirth expenses were excluded from the calculations, for example, the values of DAMC would be 3.6 for white male infants, 2.9 for white female infants, 17.4 for black male infants, and 17.5 for black female infants.)

Second, these estimates of DAMC focus only on the efficacy of increased medical care spending in reducing mortality rates. No calculations of the benefits to society from averting a death are considered. Although the question of the value of a life is clearly beyond the scope of this study, it is clear that an infant death averted generates more years of additional life than an elderly person's death averted.

4. THE "NEED" FOR ADDITIONAL PHYSICIANS

This section illustrates the use of the health production function to determine the need for additional physicians at the county level. It is assumed that the policy objective is to lower cohort-specific mortality rates in counties to the point where no mortality rate exceeds its national average in 1970. Two variants of the policy are simulated. One assumes that no physicians can be moved from existing locations. Thus, mortality rate reductions are achieved by adding new physicians to relatively high mortality rate counties. The other policy variant permits physician redistribution from low to high mortality counties. In effect, the implicit goal of the second variant is to equalize cohort-specific mortality rates across counties.

Since the final health production function estimates measured medical care in terms of expenditures rather than physicians, this simulation must be carried out in two steps. In the first, the required change in medical care expenditures for each cohort is computed using equation 8.2. In the second step, required total additional medical care expenditure is transformed into required additional physicians using the parameters of a simple regression between total medical expenditures and total physicians across counties. The results are reported as equations (8.4)–(8.5a). Both linear and logarithmic functional forms were applied to county data weighted by the inverse of the square root of the county's population.[16] Equations were estimated both for total active nonfederal patient care physicians and primary care physicians (general practitioners, medical specialists, and osteopaths).

All parameters were statistically significant at the .999 level of confidence. The linear forms of the equations, (8.4) and (8.5), are used to compute the required numbers of physicians in counties which have no physicians, since the logarithmic specifications are not defined for PC or MD = 0. The logarithmic specifications, which have slightly greater explanatory power, are used for all other counties. The formulas for the number of required additional of physicians, MD*, are given by equation (8.6), where MC* is the desired change in expenditures.

$$MC = 8.801 + (87.096 \cdot MD) \qquad R^2 = .653 \qquad (8.4)$$

$$\ln(MC) = 4.158 + (0.515 \cdot \ln(MD)) \qquad R^2 = .685 \qquad (8.4a)$$

$$MC = 0.347 + (274.358 \cdot PC) \qquad R^2 = .616 \qquad (8.5)$$

$$\ln(MC) = 4.777 + (0.666 \cdot \ln(PC)) \qquad R^2 = .660 \qquad (8.5a)$$

where

MC = estimated total medical expenditures

MD = active, nonfederal, patient care physicians

PC = active, nonfederal, primary care physicians

$$MD^* = \begin{cases} MC^*/87.096 & \text{, if } MD = 0. \\ (MC^* \cdot MD)/(.515 \cdot MC), & \text{if } MD > 0. \end{cases} \qquad (8.6)$$

Before reporting the estimates of needed physicians, it is interesting to note two implications of the medical expenditure regressions. First, recall that in chapter 6, which reported the health production functions for the infant cohorts, elasticities were reported for both medical care expenditures and measures of the relevant physician stocks (pediatricians and obstetricians). By rearranging the definition of elasticity and using the estimated values from chapter 6, an estimate of the elasticity of medical care expenditures with respect to an increase in the number of physicians can be derived by solving (8.7a) and (8.7b) for the expression given by (8.8)

$$(\Delta D/D) \approx -0.14 \cdot (\Delta MC/MC) \qquad (8.7a)$$
$$(MC = \text{medical care expenditures per}$$
$$\text{"infant")}$$

$$(\Delta D/D) \approx -0.07 \cdot (\Delta MD/MD) \qquad (8.7b)$$
$$(MD = \text{physicians per 1,000 births})$$

$$(\Delta MC/MC)/(\Delta MD/MD) \approx 0.5, \qquad (8.8)$$

where $(\Delta D/D)$ is the percentage change in the infant mortality rate. The value of the elasticity of medical care expenditures with respect to the supply of physicians computed in equation (8.8) is almost exactly the same as the elasticity estimate obtained in equation (8.4a). Since this equation was estimated with very different data (counties, total expenditures, and total physicians) from the data used in the infant mortality regressions, the high degree of consistency reinforces both findings.

Equation (8.4a) can also be used to derive an answer to the question, "How much does an additional physician add to medical care spending?" Using 1970 data, the estimate derived from (8.4a) is $95,372. (The estimate from equation (8.4) is $87,096.) This is of interest only in contrast to the oft-quoted statement that every additional physician adds about $250,000 to total medical spending. Which estimate is closer to the truth will not be evaluated here. The divergence between the two suggests how widely estimates can vary and the importance of establishing valid theoretical and empirical foundations for any such estimate.

Turning to the question of how many physicians are needed to reach a mortality rate target, table 38 reports the results of the simulation of the two policies for various groups of counties. Counties are grouped according to the percentage change in the total number of physicians. Part A of the table assumes that physicians can only be added to counties, that is, no county can lose an existing physician through reallocation. Part B shows data for counties under the assumption that physicians can be reallocated costlessly. The columns of the table indicate the average number of physicians currently in the county, the change in the number of physicians under the two policies, and several other county characteristics: the population-to-physician ratio, total population, the mortality rate (for the cohorts analyzed in this study), Medicare expenditures per enrollee, the use-need ratio (the ratio of Medicare expenditures per enrollee to the mortality rate), the value of DAMC (deaths averted per $100,000 increase in medical care spending), income per capita in 1972, percentage black population, and percentage urban population. (Except for income per capita, all data are for 1970.)

Comparing the aggregate implications of the two policies reveals a striking difference in the national need for physicians. Implementing policy A, which does not permit currently practicing physicians to be reallocated, would require adding more than 137,000 practicing physicians to the 1970 total stock of 247,588 active, nonfederal patient care physicians—a 55 percent increase. If physicians could be reallocated and if the goal were to equalize cohort-specific mortality rates across counties, then many fewer physicians would be needed; 11,800, which would be just under a 5 percent increase over the total stock.

It must be emphasized of course that the two policies do not have identical objectives. Policy A would reduce aggregate mortality, since all high-mortality areas would receive additional resources while low-mortality areas would continue to use medical care at existing rates. Under policy B, reduced mortality rates in counties which gain physicians would be offset to some extent by higher mortality rates in counties which lose physicians due to reallocation. Thus, the aggregate improvement in mortality rates would not be as great as under policy A.

In reality, the number of active, nonfederal patient care physicians in-

TABLE 38
Characteristics of Counties under Two Simulations of the Need for Physicians

Counties Grouped by Percentage Change in Number of MDs[a]

Group	No.	Percentage	Current No. of MDs[a] per county	Change in the no. of MDs[a]	Population per MD[a]	Population
Part A—Net Additions to the Physician Stock Only (Policy A)						
No change	556	18	38.6	0.0	1,927.2	33,699.5
0–25 percent increase	777	25	104.7	12.5	2,186.5	83,044.4
25–50 percent increase	560	18	69.6	25.1	2,116.5	60,673.6
50–75 percent increase	393	13	78.8	48.2	2,250.4	68,311.2
75–100 percent increase	291	10	90.6	75.0	2,093.6	58,941.9
More than 100 percent increase	491	16	99.1	147.9	1,714.4	68,754.8
Total	3,068	100	247,588.0	137,159.2	—	—
Average, all counties	—	—	80.7	44.7	2,050.6	63,567.9
Part B—Costless Reallocation of All Physicians (Policy B)						
100 percent decrease	615	19	76.0	−76.0	1742.3	65,715.6
75–100 percent decrease	187	6	83.6	−71.3	2157.7	67,092.0
50–75 percent decrease	229	8	105.1	−66.8	1975.3	83,257.2
25–50 percent decrease	282	9	59.2	−22.3	2260.1	53,403.5
0–25 percent decrease	352	12	83.5	−14.2	2321.3	65,492.0
0–25 percent increase	325	11	48.5	6.5	2249.9	47,234.5
25–50 percent increase	248	8	91.8	34.8	2258.7	69,656.0
50–75 percent increase	238	8	102.6	65.2	2295.5	61,360.5
75–100 percent increase	194	6	50.6	44.5	2059.5	47,889.7
More than 100 percent increase	398	13	106.7	159.4	1688.7	71,276.6
Total	3,068	100	247,588.0	11,794.2	—	—
Average, all counties	—	—	80.7	3.9	2050.6	63567.9

TABLE 38 (cont'd)

Counties Grouped by Percentage Change in Number of MDs[a]			Unadjusted Mortality Rate	Medicare Expends. Per Enrollee ($)	USENEED[c]	DAMC[d]	1972 Income per Capita ($)	Percentage Black Population	Percentage Urban Population
Group	No.	Percentage							
PART A—NET ADDITIONS TO THE PHYSICIAN STOCK ONLY (POLICY A)									
No change	556	18	24.8	276.4	11.5	1.16	2,997.0	3.7	24.5
0–25 percent increase	777	25	26.7	273.9	10.5	1.26	3,048.2	9.0	39.0
25–50 percent increase	560	18	27.9	273.8	10.0	1.33	3,021.1	10.8	36.2
50–75 percent increase	393	13	29.0	264.2	9.3	1.45	2,974.9	11.5	34.6
75–100 percent increase	291	10	30.1	270.2	9.1	1.45	2,975.0	11.5	34.6
More than 100 percent increase	491	16	31.7	268.0	8.5	1.52	2,915.5	10.3	36.3
Total	3068	100	—	—	—	—	—	—	—
Average, all counties	—	—	28.0	271.8	10.0	1.34	2,996.4	9.1	34.5

PART B—COSTLESS REALLOCATION OF ALL PHYSICIANS (POLICY B)

100 percent decrease	615	19	24.8	275.4	11.4	1.17	3,073.0	7.4	36.6
75–100 percent decrease	187	6	26.1	278.2	10.8	1.22	3,031.0	7.8	37.4
50–75 percent decrease	229	8	26.8	273.7	10.4	1.25	3,069.8	7.5	39.0
25–50 percent decrease	282	9	27.4	266.6	9.9	1.32	2,995.6	8.4	34.3
0–25 percent decrease	352	12	27.1	272.6	10.3	1.32	3,002.6	9.9	29.5
0–25 percent increase	325	11	28.6	269.4	9.7	1.39	2,992.3	10.6	32.6
25–50 percent increase	248	8	29.5	277.3	9.5	1.38	2,982.9	10.3	32.7
50–75 percent increase	238	8	29.7	269.7	9.2	1.45	3,000.2	11.1	32.6
75–100 percent increase	194	6	30.7	260.6	8.5	1.52	2,916.5	11.8	32.6
More than 100 percent increase	398	13	32.0	270.6	8.5	1.51	2,920.4	8.8	36.3
Total	3068	100	—	—	—	—	—	—	—
Average, all counties	—	—	28.0	271.8	10.0	1.34	2,996.4	9.1	34.5

a. MD = active, nonfederal patient care physicians.
b. Study cohorts only.
c. Ratio of Medicare expenditures per enrollee to the mortality rate (for the study cohorts).
d. DAMC = deaths averted per $100,000 increase in medical care spending (see section 2 above).

creased by about 100,000 physicians between 1970 and 1979. This corresponds to roughly a 25 percent increase in the number of such physicians per 100,000 civilian population. Over this same period the national mortality rate decreased by 9.5 percent, from 9.5 deaths per 1,000 people to 8.6 deaths per 1,000 people. Based on the health production function estimates, it is plausible to assume that the mortality rate decreases by about −0.8 percent for a 10 percent increase in the number of physicians per 100,000 population. Applying this estimate to the actual increase in physician supply over the last 10 years suggests that increased physician supply is responsible for about 20 percent of the decrease in the national mortality rate between 1970 and 1979.

Perhaps more interesting than the aggregate implications of these simulations is the comparison of characteristics of counties which would be gainers and losers under the two policies. Under policy A, how do adequately served counties which would receive no additional physicians compare to those which would be large gainers, that is, more than double their existing supply? From table 38, part A, it is easy to see that the adequately served counties have the lowest average mortality rates (24.8 deaths per 1,000 people), the highest average Medicare expenditures per enrollee ($276), the highest use-need ratio (11.5), the smallest value of DAMC, deaths averted per 100,000 increase in medical care spending (1.2), the smallest average population (33,699), the lowest percentage black population (3.7), the lowest percentage urban population (24.5), the smallest average number of physicians (38.6), and the second smallest value of population per physician (1,927).

As might be expected, the most needy counties differ dramatically. They have the highest mortality rate (31.7 deaths per 1,000 people), the second lowest level of Medicare expenditures per enrollee ($268), the lowest use-need ratio (8.5), the largest value of DAMC (1.5), the second largest average population (68,755), a much larger percentage black population (10.3), the highest percentage urban population (36.3), the second largest average number of physicians (99.1), and the smallest number of people per physician (1,714).

Comparing adequately served and most needy counties under policy B reveals essentially the same pattern for three variables, the mortality rate, USENEED, and DAMC. For several other variables, population per physician, total population, percentage black population, and percentage urban population, the most needy and least needy counties seem fairly similar. A possible explanation of this paradox is that the least needy counties include a number of areas with large populations and extremes of income and racial distributions, for example, an inner city area with a poor (predominantly black) population surrounded by or adjoining affluent, predominantly white neighborhoods and suburbs. Since the policy B simulation sums over all cohorts in a county, the favorable health experience of the numerically larger white population outweighs that of the smaller black population. Thus, the net result is a loss of physicians. Under policy A, however, only cohorts with higher than average mortality rates are included. Thus, the same county can become a relatively large net gainer of additional physicians.

Table 39 reports the distributions of counties under each policy by county size classification. Under policy A, the average number of additional physicians increases monotonically with population size. The two county groupings with the largest populations receive more than half of all new physicians, while the two smallest groups, which make up about half of all counties, receive only about 5 percent of the new physicians. Conversely, under policy B the change in the number of physicians fluctuates with population size. SMSA counties in the two largest size categories still gain the most additional physicians. However, smaller counties in SMSAs (classes 6 and 7) lose the largest numbers of physicians, about 18 percent of their physicians. The smallest counties are virtually unaffected on average (although there may be substantial redistribution within a size classification). From this perspective, then, it would appear that the largest counties would benefit the most from both policies.

Finally, what are the effects of these policies on the distribution of physicians by census division? Table 40 presents the distributions, by census division and region, of counties which are either major gainers (100 percent or larger increase in the number of physicians) or major losers (100 percent decrease) under the two policies. Also shown are the current number of physicians in these counties and the changes in the numbers of physicians under the two policies. Probably the most striking inference to be drawn from this table is that the major effect of both policies would be to alter physician distribution in favor of the northeast and north central regions. Under policy A, these two regions would receive 71 percent of the additional physicians allocated to the most needy counties. Since the two regions account for only 55 percent of all most needy counties, it is clear that the counties in these two regions are larger in population, on average, than those in the other two regions. (The average number of current physicians per county is 132, compared to an average of 59 physicians per county for the south and west regions.)

5. A COMPARISON OF THREE PROHEALTH POLICIES

Section 2 of this chapter calculated the national value of DAMC to be 1.21 deaths averted per $100,000 increase in medical care spending. In-

TABLE 39

Distribution of Counties by Population Size and the Need for Physicians under Two Policies, All Counties, 1970

Population Size Group[a]	No. of Counties[b]	Current No. of MDs[c]		Absolute Change in No. of MDs[c]				Percentage Change in Total No. of MDs[c]	
				Policy A[d]		Policy B[e]		Policy A[d]	Policy B[e]
		Total	Average	Total	Average	Total	Average		
1	799	2,215	2.8	900	1.1	36	0.1	40.6	1.6
2	927	7,992	8.6	3,924	4.2	−400	−0.4	49.1	−5.0
3	459	11,059	24.1	7,017	15.3	1,430	3.1	63.5	12.9
4	222	13,885	62.5	9,321	42.0	2,727	12.3	67.1	19.6
5	46	3,682	80.0	2,800	60.9	1,459	31.7	76.0	39.6
6	316	43,868	138.8	19,042	60.3	−7,373	−23.3	43.4	−16.8
7	127	34,370	270.6	13,798	108.7	−6,086	−47.9	40.1	−17.7
8	158	94,614	598.8	59,889	379.0	10,018	63.4	63.3	10.6
9	11	36,028	3,275.3	20,464	1,860.4	9,810	891.8	56.8	27.2

a. American Medical Association definitions:
   1 = Nonmetropolitan counties with 0 to 9,999 inhabitants.
   2 = Nonmetropolitan counties with 10,000 to 24,999 inhabitants.
   3 = Nonmetropolitan counties with 25,000 to 49,999 inhabitants.
   4 = Nonmetropolitan counties with 50,000 or more inhabitants.
   5 = Potential SMSAs.
   6 = SMSA counties with 50,000 to 499,000 inhabitants.
   7 = SMSA counties with 500,000 to 999,999 inhabitants.
   8 = SMSA counties with 1,000,000 to 4,999,999 inhabitants.
   9 = SMSA counties with 5,000,000 or more inhabitants.

b. Excludes 13 counties with missing data or no AMA classification codes.
c. Active, nonfederal patient care physicians.
d. Net additions only.
e. Costless reallocation of physicians.

TABLE 40

PERCENTAGE DISTRIBUTION OF COUNTIES AND PHYSICIANS BY MAJOR GAINS AND LOSSES OF PHYSICIANS, CENSUS DIVISIONS AND REGIONS UNDER TWO PHYSICIAN REDISTRIBUTION POLICIES, 1970

	NET ADDITIONS ONLY (POLICY A)					COSTLESS REALLOCATION OF PHYSICIANS (POLICY B)				
	No Change in MDs (n = 556)		100+ % Increase in MDs (n = 491)			100% Decrease in MDs (n = 615)		100+ % Increase in MDs (n = 398)		
	Counties (%)	Current MDs (#)	Counties (%)	Current MDs (#)	Additional MDs (#)	Counties (%)	MDs (#)	Counties (%)	Current MDs (#)	Additional MDs (#)
Census Division										
New England	0.6	2,550	5.0	4,362	7,988	0.7	1,483	5.3	4,085	7,419
Mid-Atlantic	0.4	182	14.4	16,044	23,111	1.1	2,886	16.1	13,004	19,483
South Atlantic	8.4	697	26.4	7,328	11,566	15.5	11,850	23.1	5,674	9,393
East South Central	3.3	71	9.9	807	1,223	7.4	1,078	10.6	728	1,110
West South Central	20.7	1,076	4.0	1,746	13,097	24.1	3,249	4.3	1,717	3,001
East North Central	3.6	1,123	24.6	12,147	14,626	5.7	4,492	23.4	11,231	13,457
West North Central	35.0	3,637	10.9	3,064	5,980	26.6	5,063	12.3	2,885	5,438
Mountain	21.2	2,025	3.4	161	286	11.4	4,765	3.8	136	251
Pacific	7.0	10,111	1.2	3,003	4,739	7.2	11,840	1.3	3,003	3,899
Total	100.00	21,472	100.0	48,662	72,620	100.0	46,706	100.0	42,463	63,445
Census Region										
Northeast	1.0	2,732	19.4	20,406	31,099	1.8	4,369	21.4	17,089	26,905
South	32.4	1,844	40.3	9,881	15,886	47.0	16,177	38.0	8,119	13,504
North Central	38.6	4,760	35.5	15,211	20,606	38.0	9,555	35.7	14,116	18,895
West	28.2	12,136	4.6	3,164	5,025	18.6	16,605	5.1	3,139	4,150

verting this ratio implies that the cost of each death averted is approximately $85,000. This section makes similar calculations for two other policies which could be directed at improving the nation's health: reducing cigarette consumption by 10 percent and increasing family incomes by 10 percent. Since government policy cannot simultaneously increase all families' incomes through transfer payments, we assume that this policy is directed only at persons whose family incomes were less than $10,000 in 1970. These families plus unrelated individuals contained 56 percent of the population.[17] Thus, the policy amounts to a transfer of income from the richer half of the population to the poorer half. As previously, these calculations require making several simplifying assumptions. Thus, not too much emphasis should be placed on the exact estimates of each policy's effectiveness. Of greater interest at this point are the relative magnitudes of the different estimates rather than their exact values.

The assessment of a reduced cigarette consumption policy will be based upon the experience of the antismoking campaign which began in the late 1960s and ran through 1971. Three pieces of information are required: the impact of the campaign on cigarette consumption, its cost, and cohort-specific estimates of per capita cigarette consumption. (This assessment does not take account of changes in the tar and nicotine content of cigarettes, nor does it say anything about the specific mechanisms which tie smoking to health.)

Studies by Warner and Hamilton have estimated cigarette demand functions which include estimates of the impact of antismoking advertising on per capita cigarette consumption.[18] Hamilton's equation, which held price, income, and prosmoking advertising constant, implied that the 1968–1971 antismoking campaign reduced consumption by 10 percent.[19] Warner's estimate is lower, about 4 percent, but this may be due to his omission of a prosmoking advertising variable.[20] If the omitted variable is positively related to both cigarette consumption and the amount of antismoking advertising, then the estimate of the latter's impact will be biased toward zero.[21] Consequently, the calculations reported here will assume that the desired reduction in smoking, 10 percent, can be obtained by a campaign similar to that of the 1968–1971 period.

The major cost of the antismoking campaign was the value of free media time contributed by television and radio stations under the Federal Communication Commission's fairness doctrine. This was estimated to have been worth about $75 million per year (in 1970 dollars).[22] (Prosmoking advertising was about three times as great.) Estimates of the cost of other components of the campaign, such as nonbroadcast advertising and educational seminars or lectures, are not available. For the sake of simplicity, however, it will be assumed that additional costs were $25 million, so that for the purpose of this simulation the total cost of the policy is $100 million per year. (As will be shown, the assumptions regarding the cost of the policy and its impact on cigarette consumption can be readily altered.)

Data on the distribution of smokers by sex, age, and the number of cigarettes smoked per day are obtained from the 1970 Health Interview Survey.[23] These data were used to estimate total annual consumption for each of the age-sex groups in this analysis. (Smoking by females, aged 17 to 44, was associated with the impact of cigarette consumption on infant mortality.) Total consumption for each age-sex cohort was then allocated between blacks and whites on the basis of 1978 data on cigarette smoking by race and age.[24] Total consumption for each age-sex-race group was then divided by the total population for that cohort to obtain national, cohort-specific estimates of per capita cigarette consumption. Table 41 reports the coefficients of the cigarette consumption variable from the health production function and the estimates of per capita consumption levels.

Applying equation (8.1) to these data results in an estimate of 11,215 deaths averted per year as the result of a permanent 10 percent decrease in per capita cigarette consumption. White males over the age of 44 account for more than 7,000 of these deaths, with middle-aged black males and white females contributing another 2,500 deaths to the total. Combining

TABLE 41

HEALTH PRODUCTION FUNCTION COEFFICIENTS AND AVERAGE VALUES OF PER CAPITA CIGARETTE CONSUMPTION ESTIMATES BY COHORT

COHORT	PRODUCTION FUNCTION COEFFICIENT		ANNUAL CIGARETTES CONSUMED PER CAPITA	
	Whites	Blacks	Whites	Blacks
Males				
Infants	.0027[b]	.0027[b]	2,283[a]	1,387[a]
45 to 64	.0055	.0086	3,716	3,338
65+	.0027	.0006	1,636	1,547
Females				
Infants	.0031[b]	.0011[b]	2,283[a]	1,387[a]
45 to 64	.0045	.0043	2,577	2,103
65+	.0023	.0020	796	767

a. Per capita consumption estimates are for females, aged 17 to 44.
b. From regressions not reported.

the estimated number of deaths averted with the assumed cost of the policy produces an estimate of the cost per death averted of just under $9,000.

Doubling the cost of the program, halving the assumed impact on cigarette consumption, or halving the estimate of the number of deaths averted would double the cost per death averted. If all three of these assumptions were changed at the same time, then the cost per death averted would be about $72,000. Under these conditions, the policy of reducing cigarette consumption by 10 percent would be fairly comparable to the policy of increasing medical care use by 10 percent.

Calculating the cost of reducing mortality rates by an income transfer policy is more complicated because of the greater uncertainty about the relationship between income and mortality. In particular, as was shown in chapter 7, different components of income have different effects and the magnitude of the effect depends on whether education is included in the production function specification. These calculations will be based on the coefficients of total family income (TFI), since this is the most comprehensive of the income variables used. However, two sets of estimates of the number of deaths averted will be reported—one based on TFI's coefficients with education included in the model and the other based on coefficients with education excluded. These estimates should bracket the true effect.

Table 42 reports the two sets of coefficients and the average levels of total family income for each cohort. Applying equation (8.1) to these data produces estimates of the number of deaths averted for all cohorts of 5,282 and 8,434, depending on whether education is included or excluded from the health production function. For simplicity, the remaining calculations will be based on the simple average of these two estimates, 6,858 deaths averted.

In order to compute the cost of the income transfer policy, it is necessary to estimate the aggregate income of families and unrelated individuals with total money income less than $10,000. This figure was $153 billion for families and approximately $49 billion for unrelated individuals.[25] The total of $202 billion represented 25 percent of the total national income. Thus, the cost of a 10 percent increase in total family income for persons with family incomes less than $10,000 would be about $20.2 billion.

Finally, the estimate of the cost per death averted requires determining what share of the total number of deaths averted should be allocated to persons with a family income of less than $10,000. For simplicity, it will be assumed that the coefficients of TFI in the health production function are

TABLE 42

HEALTH PRODUCTION FUNCTION COEFFICIENTS AND AVERAGE VALUES OF TOTAL FAMILY INCOME BY COHORT

| | PRODUCTION FUNCTION COEFFICIENT | | | | AVERAGE TOTAL FAMILY INCOME | |
| | WHITES | | BLACKS | | | |
Cohort	Education Included	Education Excluded	Education Included	Education Excluded	Whites	Blacks
Males						
Infants	−.0016	−.0021	−.0007	−.0011	$11,691[a]	$6,821[a]
45 to 64	−.0006	−.0011	−.0016	−.0016	11,791	7,277
65+	−.0003	−.0003	−.0003	−.0004	6,569	3,937
Females						
Infants	−.0019	−.0026	−.0023	−.0029	11,691[a]	6,821[a]
45 to 64	−.0003	−.0002	.0003	.0000	10,376	6,718
65+	.0000	−.0004	−.0003	−.0005	5,863	3,720

a. Total family incomes of females, ages 15 to 44.

independent of income. Consequently, 56 percent of the deaths averted should be allocated to the target population. Combining these various data yields a cost of almost $3 million per death averted.

The goal of this section was to compare the relative efficiency of three alternative policies for lowering mortality rates—increasing medical care consumption by 10 percent, reducing cigarette consumption by 10 percent, and increasing family incomes by 10 percent. The first policy is directed at all people in the population cohorts included in this study, the second at the entire adult population, and the third at all people with total family incomes less than $10,000. Relative efficiency is gauged by computing the cost per death averted by each of the policies. Under the most favorable set of assumptions, reducing cigarette consumption appears to be the most efficient policy, at a cost of roughly $9,000 per death averted. Increasing medical care consumption is less efficient, with a cost of approximately $85,000 per death averted, while the income transfer policy is least efficient, costing almost $3 million per death averted.

The differences in the policies' relative efficiency is striking. However, several important caveats must be stated. The first and most obvious concerns the quality of the data and the need to make a number of assumptions about the costs and impacts of the various policies. For example, changing three of the assumptions underlying the reduced cigarette consumption policy increases the estimate of the policy's cost of $72,000 per death averted. Second, the cigarette consumption simulation assumes that the effects of the antismoking campaign are permanent. To the extent that there is recidivism among those who reduce their smoking levels, then the estimate of the policy's efficiency will be overstated. Third, both the medical care subsidy and income transfer programs have goals other than reducing mortality rates. The former presumably reduces morbidity while the latter increases consumption levels of all goods (for those receiving the income transfer). Thus, focusing only on deaths averted understates the total benefits of each policy. As in the previous sections, the primary purpose of making these calculations was to illustrate how the health production function could be used to evaluate alternative policies. Definitive assessments clearly need both more recent and better quality data.

Summary

This chapter has shown how the health production function can be used to address certain policy issues. Two questions were explored. How should medical care be allocated across counties and population groups? How effective is medical care relative to other factors in reducing mortality rates?

The first question was addressed in two ways. First, it was assumed that the policy goal is to maximize the number of deaths averted for a given increase in medical care expenditures. It follows that this goal can be attained by first computing the number of deaths averted per given increase in medical spending for both areas and population groups, and then ranking them in descending order. By allocating additional funds to the area or groups with the largest values, the total number of deaths averted will be maximized.

Nationwide, it was estimated that a 10 percent increase in medical care spending would reduce the mortality rate by 1.61 percent. The total cost of the policy would be about $2.3 billion (in 1970) and almost 28,000 deaths would be averted. Together, these figures imply that 1.21 deaths are averted for each $100,000 increase in medical care spending.

Applying this criterion, which was called DAMC, to county data led to three fairly strong findings. First, DAMC is only weakly related to the ratio of population-to-physicians, the primary criterion now used to designate health manpower shortage areas. As a result, comparing the 500 counties with the greatest "need" according to the two criteria revealed that only about 20 percent of counties fall into both categories.

Second, a much higher proportion of the counties with high values of DAMC are in the southern region compared to counties with high population-to-physician ratios—82 percent of the former as opposed to 54 percent of the latter. Conversely, the DAMC criterion included far fewer counties in the north central region, only 12 percent, while 36 percent of the high population-to-physician ratio counties were in that region. The primary explanation seems to be that while many counties in the north central (and western) regions have very few physicians, they also have relatively more healthy populations and relatively higher use of services than in southern counties.

This leads to the third conclusion. DAMC has a large negative correlation of about −0.8 with a readily available indicator, the ratio of Medicare expenditures per enrollee to the mortality rate. The large negative correlation means that in counties where use relative to need tends to be high, the value of DAMC tends to be low. In effect, this correlation suggests that additional medical care resources should be allocated to areas where use is low relative to need.

Computing DAMC for the various population groups in this study revealed that the elderly tend to have larger values than the infant and middle-aged cohorts, and blacks tend to have larger values than whites.

(There was one exception to each of these statements.) These results lend support to programs which subsidize medical care use by the elderly (Medicare) and by racial minorities.

The finding of a relatively low value for infants must be qualified in two ways, however. First, the estimate of the cost of medical care for infants was probably overstated, since it included the full costs of childbirth. Some of this expense should probably be assigned to maternal care rather than infant care (for example, extra days in the hospital following caesarean delivery). Making this type of adjustment would increase the value of DAMC for infants. Second, this criterion focuses only on the costs of averting a death. It does not consider the benefits to society. This too needs to be considered when debating, for example, whether to increase the scope of the Medicare program or to establish the Child Health Assessment Program. The benefits from averting a death were not considered by this study.

The second way the resource allocation issue was approached was by asking, "How much additional medical care spending would a county need in order to reduce its cohort-specific mortality rates to some desired level?" Simulations were based on the target of reducing cohort-specific mortality rates in each county to their national averages for 1970. One simulation assumed that resources could only be added to a county, while the other permitted redistribution from one county to another. (In effect, the second approach would equalize mortality rates across counties at their 1970 national averages.)

Additional medical spending was transformed into additional physicians needed by using the parameters of a simple regression equation which related total medical care expenditures in a county to the total numbers of active, nonfederal primary care and patient care physicians. These regressions revealed that a 10 percent increase in the number of physicians would increase spending by about 5 percent.

The simulations indicated that only about 12,000 additional physicians would be needed if complete redistribution were feasible. Just over half of all counties would lose some physicians. However, if the policy could only add physicians to locations, then the number needed would be much larger, approximately 137,000 physicians. All but 18 percent of counties would receive some additional physicians.

The percentage change in a county's supply of physicians was strongly related to the mortality rate, the use-need ratio, and the value of DAMC. Under both policy simulations, the majority of additional physicians are allocated to counties with the largest populations. Counties which lose physicians tend to be smaller counties in SMSAs. Nonmetropolitan counties, particularly those in the smallest population category, are largely un-affected by the redistribution schemes.

The simulations also suggested that additional physicians would be added primarily to the northeast and north central regions. Under policy B, which permits physician reallocation, the West would be the primary loser of physicians. In contrast, identifying shortage areas on the basis of the value of DAMC would provide additional resources primarily to the South. The difference between the two sets of implications is explained by the fact that the underlying policies have different objectives. One at-tempts to maximize the number of deaths averted, given a fixed budget. The other sets a particular mortality rate reduction as its target, regard-less of the cost of the policy.

Finally, the general question of how expanding medical care use com-pares to other possible policies for reducing mortality rates was evaluated by computing the cost per death averted for three alternative policies: in-creasing medical care expenditures by 10 percent; reducing per capita cigarette consumption by 10 percent; and increasing total family income by 10 percent for persons in families and unrelated individuals with total money incomes less than $10,000 in 1970. Inadequate data and missing information required making a number of strong assumptions. Thus, the specific estimates of the cost per death averted under the three policies are not likely to be highly reliable. Nevertheless, the estimates differed by several orders of magnitude, suggesting that an ordinal ranking would probably not be altered if the costs were recomputed with better data. In particular, it was found that reducing cigarette consumption was the most efficient of the three, followed by increasing medical care consumption, and increasing incomes of lower-income persons.

In reporting these implications, it must be emphasized that the primary goal of this chapter has been to illustrate the usefulness of the health pro-duction function for evaluating policy issues. The specific implications should not necessarily be applied to current policy problems. The data used by this study are now more than 10 years old and may not reflect cur-rent conditions very well. What these simulations do suggest for current use is that (1) the ratio of population to physicians may not be a very good criterion for identifying shortage areas; (2) the ratio of Medicare expen-ditures per enrollee to the mortality rate appears to be a better indicator of underservice; (3) this ratio would be more useful if Medicare expenditures were available by sex and race; and (4) data on expenditures per capita for other population cohorts would also be very useful.

9

SUMMARY AND CONCLUSIONS

Three broad questions motivated the analyses undertaken by this study. What is the relationship between medical care use and various mortality rates? How do income and education influence mortality rates? Do the medical care-mortality relationships have any implications for the distribution of medical care in general and physicians in particular?

The study's primary analytic task has been the specification and estimation of a series of age-sex-race-specific health production functions. Health was measured by an inverse indicator, the cohort-specific mortality rate. The health production function was shown to be part of a more complete model of the demand for and the supply of health. The main implication (for this study) of the broader model is that the demand for medical care and the production of health are jointly determined variables, that is, medical care use affects health, but health also influences the amount of medical care use. (This simultaneous relationship has direct implications for the statistical methods used.) In addition, reference was made to several taxonomic theories of health in order to help classify potential independent variables into four broad groups: medical care use, lifestyle/ behavior, heredity or genetic stock, and environment. For the analysis of infant mortality, the last three factors were grouped into a single set of variables designed to measure risk at birth.

The geographic unit of analysis for the study was the county group, as defined by the Bureau of the Census. A county group consists of one or more whole counties with a minimum population of 250,000 people. The criteria for grouping counties are similar to those used to designate state economic areas. However, a county group can encompass counties in more than one state. In 1970, there were 407 county groups and county group subareas (individual counties of more than 250,000 people within a county group).

County-level mortality and population data were obtained from a special study supported by the National Center for Health Statistics. These data, which span the years 1968 to 1972, were aggregated and averaged to form age-sex-race-specific mortality rates for each county group. The population groups analyzed consisted of the following eight adult cohorts and four infant cohorts:

> White males, 45 to 64 years old
> Black males, 45 to 64 years old
> White females, 45 to 64 years old
> Black females, 45 to 64 years old
> White males, 65 and older
> Black males, 65 and older
> White females, 65 and older
> Black females, 65 and older
> White male infants (less than 1 year old)
> Black male infants (less than 1 year old)
> White female infants (less than 1 year old)
> Black female infants (less than 1 year old)

For the adult cohorts, separate production functions were estimated for several groupings of deaths: all causes, all natural causes, all external causes, all cancers, all cardiovascular diseases, and ischemic heart diseases. Infant deaths were grouped into neonatal and postneonatal mortalities, as well as infant mortalities.

Other data for 1970 were obtained from a number of sources. The primary one was a 2 percent sample of the 1970 Census of Population. These data permitted the construction of a number of important socio-demographic variables (e.g., income, education, marital and family status, occupation, labor force participation, race, age, sex, nativity, and migration) for each of the study cohorts. (Data for women of childbearing age, 14 to 44, were used in the infant mortality analysis.)

Three approaches to measuring medical care use were investigated: the ratios of physicians, nurses, and acute care hospital beds per 1,000 people in the county group, cohort-specific estimates of these ratios, and Medicare expenditures per enrollee in the county group. On both theoretical and empirical grounds, Medicare expenditures per enrollee proved to be the best measure of medical care use. Consequently, the statistical results are based primarily on the use of that variable in the health production functions. (In the infant mortality analysis, variables measuring the numbers of obstetricians and pediatricians per 1,000 live births performed about as well, and in some cases better, than Medicare expenditures per enrollee.)

The next section of this chapter summarizes the study's principal findings. The last section draws some tentative conclusions and makes suggestions for further research.

Summary of Findings

The primary question underlying this study is "Does greater medical care use contribute to significantly lower mortality rates?" Based on estimates from the health production functions, which hold fixed the effects of a number of sociodemographic, behavioral, and environmental factors, the answer is an unambiguous, "Yes." Except for middle-aged males, the estimates suggest that a 10 percent increase in per capita medical care use is associated with about a 1.5 percent decrease in mortality rates. This result was obtained for the four infant cohorts, for all adult female cohorts, and for elderly (65 and older) male cohorts. Increased medical care use appears to have about twice as large an impact on white, middle-aged (45 to 64 years old) males and about half as large an impact on black, middle-aged males as on the other cohorts. The reasons for these two divergences are not explored in this study.

Analysis of cause-specific mortality rates revealed a pattern of medical care effects consistent with both the general finding and with impressionistic evidence of the diagnostic conditions medical care can effectively treat. In particular, medical care use generally had no significant impact on deaths from cancers and from external causes. Between 1960 and 1970, mortality rates for these two causes of death showed no downward trend. However, deaths from ischemic heart disease and from all cardiovascular causes were generally more sensitive to medical care use than deaths from all causes, particularly for white males. Mortality rates from this group of diseases have been declining sharply since 1960.

The analysis of the relationship between education, income, and mortality rates revealed that education has a consistently negative association with mortality rates. Numerous other studies have had the same result. The relationship between income and mortality rates, however, appears to be much more complex. Total family income has a generally negative effect on mortality rates. For infants, the impact of total family income is statistically significant for three of four cohorts and has a moderate elasticity: a 10 percent increase in income would lower infant mortality by between 1.6 and 2.2 percent (except for black male infants). For adults, the effect of total family income is statistically significant for only two cohorts and generally has a very small quantitative impact on mortality.

The explanation of this seemingly tenuous relationship appears to lie in the fact that different types of income have different effects on mortality rates. In particular, nonlabor income from either public welfare programs or private sources (rents, dividends, private pensions, etc.) has a consistently negative and generally statistically significant effect. In fact, for some cohorts a 10 percent increase in private transfer payments, which make up only a small proportion of total income, has a quantitatively larger impact on mortality than a 10 percent increase in total income. The impact of income from earnings, however, depends on the age of the cohort. For working age cohorts (45 to 64 years old), earned income has a generally negative effect—higher earned income is associated with lower mortality rates. For elderly cohorts (65 and older), earned income has a generally positive effect. Income from all nonlabor sources (including other family members) shows the opposite signs. This pattern seems to imply that for persons of working age, higher earned income probably reflects greater command over resources and better health. Conversely, for people of retirement age, higher earned income may reflect a greater need to work, that is, lower economic status, as well as the possibly deleterious effects of work itself on the health of the elderly.

Finally, health production function parameter estimates were applied to several policy questions, both to identify the estimates' implications for policy and to illustrate how the health production function could be used in the policy process. The issues explored were the allocation of medical care resources among both geographic areas and population groups, and the relative efficiency of increasing medical care use as a policy for reducing mortality rates. The impact on mortality rates of increasing medical care use was compared to two alternative policies: reducing cigarette consumption and increasing income transfers to low-income families and individuals. These policy comparisons took account of the cost of each policy as well as its effect on mortality rates.

The geographic distribution issue was addressed in two ways in order to demonstrate how differences in the goal of a policy can influence the allocation of resources. In one case, the goal was to maximize the number of lives saved (more precisely, deaths averted) by a 10 percent increase in per capita medical care spending. In the other case, the policy's goal was to reduce above-average, cohort-specific mortality rates to their national average in 1970. The first policy aims to maximize the health outcome for a given budget, while the second attempts to reach a predetermined health target without any budget constraint.

The first policy was addressed in two steps. First, the health production function parameters were used to estimate the number of deaths averted per $100,000 increase in medical care spending for each county in the nation. Second, counties were ranked on the basis of the number of deaths averted. The policy's objective, maximizing the number of deaths averted for a given increase in medical care spending, would be reached by making grants or providing additional medical resources to those counties with the largest values of the ranking criterion. Counties with successively smaller values of the ranking criterion would receive additional resources until the given budget was exhausted. This allocation scheme would maximize the number of deaths averted.

Examining the geographic distribution of the 500 counties with the largest value of the deaths averted criterion revealed that 82 percent are located in the South. In contrast to this, 53 percent of the 500 counties with the largest population-per-primary-care-physician ratios, an alternative ranking criterion, are in the South. A much higher proportion of the second group of counties is located in the north central and western regions, 47 percent, compared to only 15 percent of the 500 counties with the largest values of the deaths averted criterion. The main reason for the divergence between these two criteria seems to be that in the case of the population-per-primary-care-physician ratio, many counties which have only a few physicians also have relatively healthy populations.

One potential indicator of the use of medical care relative to the need for care is the ratio of Medicare expenditures per enrollee to the unadjusted mortality rate. The population-per-primary-care-physician ratio is only weakly correlated with both the number of deaths averted per $100,000 increase in medical care spending and the proxy use-need ratio. The last two factors, however, have a large negative correlation, approximately -0.8. This implies that in counties where the use of services relative to need is high, the payoff from additional medical care expenditures would be relatively small. The advantage of the proposed use-need indicator is that both the numerator and denominator measure characteristics of a county's residents regardless of where they might travel to obtain medical care or where death might occur. The population-per-primary-care-physician ratio does not take account of either travel patterns to obtain medical care or any indicator of a population's health.

The second policy application focused on the need for additional medical care by asking how much more medical care would be required to

reduce above average, cohort-specific mortality rates to their 1970 national average. Two variants of this policy were explored. One assumes
that physicians can only be added to an area. Thus, the goal is to reduce
mortality rates in high mortality areas without altering the supply of
physicians in low mortality areas. The other variant assumes that physicians can be reallocated costlessly. In effect, the goal of the second policy
is to equalize cohort-specific mortality rates across counties at the national
average.

The number of additional physicians needed (or required) was computed by using the health production estimates to translate the desired
change in the mortality rate into the required change in medical care expenditures. The latter was then converted into the required change in
physicians on the basis of an estimated relationship across counties between total medical care expenditures and the total supply of active,
nonfederal, patient care physicians. (This equation predicted that a 10
percent increase in the supply of physicians would increase total medical
care spending by about 5 percent. For changes of this magnitude, this
amounts to approximately $90,000 (in 1970 dollars) of additional medical
care expenditures per additional physician.)

As might be expected, the two variants had dramatically different implications for the aggregate need for additional physicians. The first implied that about 137,000 more physicians would have to be added to the
1970 stock of 247,500 active, nonfederal, patient care physicians in order
to reduce all above-average, cohort-specific mortality rates to their 1970
national averages. The second variant implied that fewer than 12,000 extra physicians would be needed to equalize cohort-specific mortality rates
across counties if physicians could be reallocated costlessly. It must be
emphasized, of course, that these variants are not identical. The first
would result in a net reduction in the national mortality rate for these
cohorts, from 26.7 deaths per thousand people to 25.3 deaths per thousand. The second would have no impact on national mortality rates.

The two policies, however, were similar in terms of their implications
for the regional distribution of physicians. Both would increase the supplies of physicians in the northeast and north central regions. Furthermore, under the second policy variant, which permits physician reallocation, the largest losses in physician supply would occur in the West, while
the South would have only a small net reduction.

The apparent reason for the difference between these policies' regional
implications and those of the first policy simulation is the difference in the
way the policies' goals were formulated. The first focused on maximizing
the number of deaths averted for a given increase in medical expenditures.

Thus, implicitly at least, the cost of medical care and the cost of averting a death are integral parts of the allocation criterion, the number of deaths averted per \$100,000 increase in medical care spending. The goal of the second policy application was simply to reduce mortality rates without regard to cost implications. Thus, it is not surprising that the South, which has lower per capita medical care expenditures than other regions, would receive the greatest benefit under the first policy, while the largest counties in the declining northeast and north central regions, which tend to have the highest medical care costs, benefit the most under the second type of policy.

The two variants of the second policy simulation also have similar implications for physician distribution across counties grouped by population size. In both cases, counties with the largest populations, more than 1,000,000 people, receive the major share of the added physicians. The smallest counties, nonmetropolitan counties with fewer than 25,000 residents, are largely unaffected. Counties which would experience the greatest decreases in physician supply (under the second variant) are small metropolitan counties with populations between 50,000 and 1,000,000 people. Thus, redistribution would take place primarily between smaller and larger metropolitan counties.

A third policy application explored the allocation of medical care resources among population cohorts. This issue was addressed in the same way as the first geographic distribution simulation. It was assumed that the policy goal is to maximize the number of deaths averted for a given medical expenditure increase. The policy question is, which population cohorts should receive priority for receiving medical care subsidies? Thus, the number of deaths averted per \$100,000 increase in spending was computed for each study cohort using the cohort-specific health production function estimates. These calculations revealed that in general, the number of deaths averted is greater for the elderly than for other age groups, and greater for blacks than for whites.

No attempt was made, however, to evaluate the benefit from averting a death in each cohort. Furthermore, the calculations for the number of infant deaths averted assumed that the full costs of prenatal care and childbirth should be allocated to the goal of reducing infant mortality, rather than split between reducing both infant and maternal mortality. Thus, these estimates tend to understate the number of infant deaths averted per \$100,000 increase in spending for reduced infant mortality.

The final policy application was a highly exploratory comparison of three alternative policies for reducing mortality rates: increasing medical care use by 10 percent; reducing cigarette consumption by 10 percent; and increasing incomes of the poorer half of the nation's population by 10 percent. (Each of these factors, medical care use, cigarette sales, and total family income was an element of the health production functions.) For each policy, the number of deaths averted per $100,000 of policy cost was computed. The inverse of this estimate, the cost per death averted, was then used to rank the three policies in terms of their relative efficiency in reducing mortality rates.

Although the calculations themselves are conceptually straightforward, it was necessary to make several strong assumptions in order to use available data. Furthermore, in no case is reducing mortality rates the only goal of the policy. Both increased medical care use and reduced cigarette consumption have reduced morbidity rates as additional goals, while income transfer policies are geared primarily toward increasing the consumption of all goods and services by the poor, not just medical care or other health contributing goods. Thus, the ranking of policies is based on an evaluation along only one of possibly several policy goals. Finally, it is assumed that each policy represents a permanent one-time change. This is particularly relevant to assessing the reduced cigarette consumption policy, since no allowance is made for recidivism by those who reduce their cigarette consumption levels.

Given these caveats, the calculations revealed that reducing cigarette consumption was the most efficient policy, with a cost per death averted of roughly $9,000. (Changing three key assumptions increased this estimate to $72,000 per death averted, however.) Increasing medical care use was estimated to cost about $85,000 per death averted. Finally, the income transfer policy is the least efficient of the three, with a cost of almost $3,000,000 per death averted.

It must be emphasized, however, that the primary purpose of these simulations was to illustrate how the health production function estimates could be used to address various policy issues. These results should not be applied to current policy problems without careful consideration. They are based on data that are more than 10 years old and, in several cases, require a number of strong assumptions about the nature of certain relationships. Rather than giving clear guidelines for current policy choices, these simulations indicate the types of data which would be needed to assess current policy issues.

Although not the primary focus of this study, the findings from the health production function for factors other than medical care, income, and education are also of interest. In general, the results conformed with prior expectations. For adults, several indirect measures of health status had the expected signs in the mortality equations. Average age, the percentage reporting activity-limiting disabilities, and the percentage not in the labor force (female cohorts only) generally had positive coefficients. Proxies for a relatively good health status, the percentage of the cohort which resided in a different state five years earlier, the number of children ever born (female cohorts only), and the percentage not currently in the labor force who last worked in 1968 or later (male cohorts only) generally had negative coefficients.

Behavior/lifestyle variables (in addition to income and education) included the percentage employed in agriculture (males only), the percentage married, cigarette sales per capita in the state, and cohort-specific excess deaths from alcoholism and cirrhosis of the liver. Both the agricultural employment and marital status variables had the expected negative relationship with mortality rates, while the other two variables were associated with higher mortality rates. The use of cigarettes sold per capita in the state as a proxy for actual consumption was reinforced by this variable's coefficients in the cause-specific mortality analysis. In particular, the coefficients were usually largest in magnitude, positive, and statistically significant in the ischemic heart and cardiovascular disease equations (for all but two cohorts—elderly females). Conversely, all coefficients but one were statistically insignificant in the equation for deaths from external causes. The coefficients in the cancer equations were positive for all male cohorts (statistically significant and larger in magnitude for the middle-aged cohorts), but statistically insignificant (and negative) for three female cohorts.

Analysis of the impact of environmental factors was limited by the lack of good quality data. Although the full set of environmental variables was generally significant as a group, interpretation of specific variables was difficult because of possible correlations with other factors. More accurate measurement of better defined variables for smaller geographic areas is needed for this type of study.

The analysis of infant mortality rates found, like many other studies, that risk at birth is clearly the most important determinant of infant mortality. Birth risk was measured by the expected mortality rate, which was computed from the county-specific distribution of births by birthweight and national sex-race-weight-specific motality rates. The expected mortality rate had a large, positive coefficient and was statistically significant in all equations. The percentage of births in hospitals also had a large impact in the postneonatal and infant mortality equations. The percentage of births to mothers of high-risk age was generally less significant. Crude estimates of the contribution of reduced risk at birth to reduced infant mortality rates over the period 1969 to 1978 indicated that reductions in risk were responsible for about one-third of the reduction in white infant mortality rates and one quarter of the reduction in black infant mortality rates. (Increased medical care use accounted for about 13 percent of the reduction for both races.)

Finally, a highly exploratory analysis was conducted of the effects on neonatal mortality rates of two major social policies of the late 1960s: Medicaid coverage of first-time pregnancies and liberalization of abortion laws. The results suggested that states which do not cover first-time pregnancies through Medicaid programs have higher neonatal mortality rates than other states. Neonatal mortality rates were lower, however, in states which had relaxed their abortion laws before 1971 or had relatively higher abortion rates (abortions per 1,000 live births).

Although these results must be considered tentative because of the crude way in which these variables were constructed, the mechanisms through which these policies influence neonatal mortality seem clear. Broader Medicaid coverage means earlier and more frequent prenatal care for eligible women. Abortion rates are higher for very young and very old women than for women of prime childbearing age, higher for single than for married women, and higher for blacks than for whites. Since each of these relationships is associated with greater risks at birth, higher abortion rates probably result in a smaller proportion of high-risk births.

Conclusions and Suggestions for Further Research

This study has presented empirical evidence which shows that greater medical care use is a significant factor explaining lower mortality rates. The magnitude of this relationship is larger than reported in earlier studies. Furthermore, the validity of this study's empirical findings is probably greater than in earlier studies because of separate estimation of the health production function for age-sex-race-specific population cohorts, the use of high quality data from the 1970 Census of Population, and more accurate measurement of the use of medical care. This last factor is particularly important since the analysis also revealed that the availability of medical care providers in an area is a poor indicator of medical care use. Most studies which have concluded that medical care does not affect mortality rates have used the availability of physicians (usually the physician-to-population ratio) as the primary measure of medical care use.

This basic result has implications for two broad policy issues. The first is that expanding medical care use should continue to be an element of effort to improve the nation's health. This is not to say that medical care use is the most important factor influencing health, or that increasing its use is the most efficient policy to follow. In fact, a crude comparison of three prohealth policies suggested that changing personal behavior, as represented by reducing cigarette consumption, is probably more efficient. The difficulty, of course, is that government efforts to change behavior raise serious political and ethical questions about interference with individual's rights and freedom of choice in a demoncratic society. On a more technical level, there are questions of what methods work and how long desired behavioral changes are likely to persist.

It is also hoped that the exploratory comparison of alternative prohealth policies has demonstrated the importance of considering a policy's costs as well as its effects on health. In particular, it is sometimes argued that policies to improve health should focus primarily on the factors which have the greatest impact on health, without much consideration of alternative policies' costs. Thus, the argument continues, because life-style and environment have a greater impact on health than does medical care, more should be spent on changing behavior and the environment than is spent on medical care. The flaw in this reasoning is that the costs of these policies are not fully considered.

Thus, this study has shown that expanding medical care use appears to satisfy a necessary condition for serious consideration as a policy option—it does have a significant impact on mortality rates. Whether the impact is large or small, or the policy useful or useless are much more complicated questions. They can be answered only in relation to the costs and effectiveness of other approaches to reducing mortality rates.

The second broad policy issue to which this study's results are pertinent is the debate over national health insurance and the question of how much medical care can the nation afford. For good reason, the greatest emphasis in recent years has been on the cost of medical care—its growing share of the gross national product, the share of government expenditures devoted to medical care, and the rate of increase in the medical care component of the Consumer Price Index. In a time of economic stagnation, these factors cannot be ignored. However, the impact of medical care on mortality rates, and on health more broadly, should also not be ignored. Better evidence on the mortality-medical care tradeoff will interject this important dimension into the debate over how much medical care the nation should have. "How much can we afford?" is a meaningless question without the answer to its companion, "What are we buying?"

Finally, on a more technical level, the study has demonstrated how the health production function concept can be used to address questions of medical care resource allocation. In particular, it was shown that the population-per-physician ratio is probably not a very good indicator of either medical underservice or the need for additional physicians. A potentially much better indicator is the ratio of Medicare expenditures per enrollee to the mortality rate. These data are readily available at the county level on an annual basis. More importantly, this ratio appears to be a good index of the use of medical care relative to the need for care.

Most of the data used in this study are more than 10 years old. Thus, it is clear that the first step in further research efforts should be replication with more recent data. Data from the 1980 Census of Population should provide an excellent opportunity to repeat much of the analysis.

The 1980 Census data offer another major research opportunity, namely, examining changes in mortality rates between 1970 and 1980. The advantage of this type of analysis is that it provides a means of holding constant many area-specific factors, such as climate and elevation, which were measured very imperfectly in the current study. At the same time, major population shifts among regions add another dimension to the cross-sectional variation observed in 1970. Finally, all areas of the country have experienced major increases in medical care expenditures over the last 10 years. Since increasing medical care use is an intertemporal rather than cross-sectional phenomenon, analysis of both 1970 and 1980 data will offer a rigorous test of the medical care-mortality hypothesis.

Lastly, this study has clearly demonstrated the need for and utility of data on medical care expenditures by age, sex, and race. Particular emphasis needs to be placed on data of all types for age groups 65 and older. This group is responsible for a disproportionate share of medical care use and expenditures. It is projected to become a larger share of the total population. In addition, the 65 and older group needs to be broken down into smaller age groupings because of major differences between people 85 and older and those between the ages of 65 and 74, and 75 and 84.

Collecting such data for all counties in the United States would clearly be an exorbitant expense. More feasible, perhaps, would be the selection of a sample of counties which is representative of the U.S. population. This sample could be used to collect both expenditure and health data on a continuing basis and would provide a natural laboratory for both cross-sectional and intertemporal analysis.

The most obvious candidate for this type of data collection is a modified version of the Health Interview Survey. In its current form, the Health Interview Survey does not regularly collect expenditure data, the 28 identified local areas are not representative of the U.S. population, and there are not enough of them for valid cross-sectional analysis. Another possibility, though less complete, is the reporting of Medicare data on a more disaggregated basis, for example, by sex, race, and age (65 to 74, 75 to 84, and 85 and older for example). Given the size of the medical care industry and the importance of good health to the nation's well-being, the investment in better data would appear to be most worthwhile.

APPENDIX A

EMPIRICAL ISSUES AND METHODS

This appendix discusses background empirical issues underlying the development and specification of the empirical model. These issues include the choice of a unit of analysis, data sources and file construction, cohort specification, choice of functional form, and methods for dealing with potential econometric problems (heteroskedasticity, specification bias, and simultaneous equation bias).

Unit of Analysis

As noted in chapter 1, the geographic unit of analysis for this study is the county group, which is defined by the Bureau of the Census.[1] The country is divided into areas and subareas, each of which has a population of 250,000 or more. County groups may cross state boundaries. Each area is an extension of the Standard Metropolitan Statistical Area (SMSA) concept—an urban center and surrounding counties tied to that center by trade and commuting patterns. In rural areas which do not contain an SMSA, the urban center is defined as a city with 20,000 to 50,000 population. Subareas within each county group are SMSAs or components of SMSAs with populations greater than 250,000 people. There were 407 identified areas and subareas in 1970.

Choosing the county group as the unit of analysis provides more observations than use of either states or SMSAs. In addition, there should be less intraarea variation in the data for a county group than for a state. At the same time, county groups provide information on rural areas, since the presence of a central city of more than 50,000 people is not required to construct a county group. Compared to individual counties, the county group contains a much larger population for analysis and is not likely to be as affected by the border-crossing problem, particularly since the county group can cross state boundaries.

Within each county group, the study population is divided into 16 adult cohorts and 4 infant cohorts. The adult population consists of four age groupings, 45 to 54, 55 to 64, 65 to 74, and 75 and older, for both sexes and two races (white and black). The infant cohorts are broken down by sex and race. The main reason for disaggregating the population in this way is to control for the effects of variations in biological and sociocultural characteristics which may be associated with age, sex, and race but are difficult to measure directly. The most obvious factor is natural changes in health stock usually associated with aging. Similarly, attitudes about health and medical care, the effects of racial discrimination, and inherited physical traits may be other factors which are difficult to observe but can be held reasonably fixed by investigating age-sex-race-specific population cohorts.

The theory developed in chapter 2 focused on the individual's decisions regarding levels of health and medical care use. As developed in chapter 2, the health production function was specified as

$$h_{ik} = h(m_{ik}, pc_{ik}, AC_k) \tag{A.1}$$

where

h_{ik} = health of the ith individual in the kth area,

m_{ik} = consumption of medical care,

pc_{ik} = other personal characteristics,

AC_k = area characteristics.

However, the function to be estimated is defined for the population cohort, that is

$$H_{jk} = H(M_{jk}, PC_{jk}, AC_k) \tag{A.2}$$

where

$$H_{jk} = \sum_{i}^{n_{jk}} h_{ik}/n_{jk} = \text{health of the } jth \text{ age-sex-race cohort in the } k\text{th area}$$

$$M_{jk} = \sum_{i}^{n_{jk}} m_{ik}/n_{jk},$$

$$PC_{jk} = \sum_i^{n_{jk}} pc_{ik}/n_{jk}, \text{ and}$$

n_{jk} = number of people in the jth cohort and kth area.

The primary advantage of aggregating individual data to the county group level is that this type of aggregation reduces much of the variation in other unobservable personal characteristics. For example, the distribution of intellectual capacity is probably more evenly distributed across geographic areas than across individuals.[2] Thus, the production function represented by equation (A.2) will be estimated initially for 16 adult cohorts and 4 infant cohorts.

Econometric Issues

Estimating the parameters of the health production function requires choosing a mathematical form for the function and an estimation method. In addition, one should determine whether bias is likely to arise from problems such as heteroskedasticity and specification error. This section discusses each of these econometric issues and describes the procedures used to deal with them.

1. CHOICE OF FUNCTIONAL FORM

The mathematical form chosen for the production function should satisfy three criteria. First, it should be flexible enough to permit a marginal product of medical care with respect to mortality rates which can assume both negative and positive signs and is sensitive to variations in local conditions. This permits testing of the hypothesis that there is a threshold beyond which the consumption of additional medical care services contributes nothing to reducing mortality rates. Second, the signs of the parameters of the medical care variables should be consistent with a priori expectations. Third, a scatter diagram of residuals should not reveal any nonrandom patterns. This generally indicates the absence of any serious specification error.

Although there are potentially many forms which meet these criteria, we shall focus on a modified version of the well-known Cobb-Douglas production function.

$$D_{ij} = AM_{ij}{}^{\alpha_j}e^{(\beta_j M_{ij} + \Sigma_s \alpha_{js} X_{ijs})}U_{ij}, \tag{A.3}$$

where

D_{ij} = mortality rate of the jth cohort in the ith county group

M_{ij} = medical care proxy

X_{ijs} = other independent variables, and

the subscripts refer to

i = 1, ..., n county groups.

j = 1, ..., k age-sex-race-specific cohorts

s = 1, ..., m independent variables.

The marginal product of medical care is represented by the expression

$$MP_{ij} = \frac{\partial D_{ij}}{\partial M_{ij}} = \frac{D_{ij}(\alpha_j + \beta_j M_{ij})}{M_{ij}} \tag{A.4}$$

Since D_{ij} could be replaced by equation (A.3), the marginal product is clearly a function of variations in local conditions. On a priori grounds, we expect $\alpha_j < 0$ and $\beta_j > 0$. This suggests that at some levels of M_{ij}, the marginal product of medical care may not be significantly different from zero, or could be positive, that is, more medical care increases mortality rates. If $\beta_j < 0$, on the other hand, then the marginal product is strictly negative (assuming $\alpha_j < 0$). Finally, the elasticity of the mortality rate with respect to medical care (the percentage change in the mortality rate for a small percentage change in medical care) is also given by a simple expression.

$$\xi_{M_{ij}} = \alpha_j + \beta_j M_{ij} \tag{A.5}$$

This functional form offers two additional advantages which justify its use. First, applying a logarithmic transformation to equation (A.3) converts it into an expression which is linear in the parameters. Thus, simple multivariate regression techniques can be applied. Second, and perhaps most important, the estimated elasticity is invariant with respect to a scalar transformation of the medical care variable. As discussed at length in chapter 4, one of the available proxy measures of medical care use is Medicare expenditures per enrollee in each county group, M_i. It was argued that it is plausible to assume that

$$M_i = \delta_j MC_{ij} \tag{A.6}$$

where MC_{ij} is cohort-specific medical care expenditures (consumption) per capita. Substituting (A.6) into (A.3), it can be shown that the elasticity of the mortality rate with respect to cohort-specific medical care expenditures per capita is

$$\xi_{MC_{ij}} = \alpha_j + \beta_j \delta_j MC_{ij} \qquad (A.7)$$

From (A.6), however, it is clear that

$$\xi_{MC_{ij}} = \alpha_j + \beta_j M_i = \xi_{M_{ij}}$$

If $\beta_j = 0$, then the elasticity is independent of local conditions (although the marginal product is not).

2. HETEROSKEDASTICITY

Heteroskedasticity, the existence of a nonconstant variance of the error term, is a common characteristic of relationships estimated with cross-sectional data. This is particularly true when the unit of analysis is a geographic entity which can vary widely in the size of its population. For this study, heteroskedasticity can arise because the stability of mortality *rates* for an area is likely to be positively correlated with the size of the underlying population. In other words, random fluctuations in mortality rates are likely to be larger for less populated areas.[3] Although heteroskedasticity does not imply biased parameter estimates, it does bias the estimated standard errors, thus invalidating the conventional tests of statistical significance.

Two tests will be performed to detect the presence of heteroskedasticity. The implicit assumption is that if the variance is not constant, it is likely to be correlated with the population of the county group. Therefore, all observations will be ranked in ascending order by population. A scatter diagram of the residuals against the sequence of observations will provide visual evidence regarding the constancy of the error term's variance.

The second test requires dividing the ordered observation set into three partitions. The mortality production function will then be estimated separately for each of the two extreme partitions. The null hypothesis of equal variances can be tested by computing an F-statistic based on the sums-of-squared residuals from the regressions on the partitioned data.[4] If these tests suggest that the error term is heteroskedastic, then the observations should be weighted by the inverse of the square root of the cohort's population in each country group. This is a standard adjustment which has been used in several other studies.[5]

3. SIMULTANEOUS EQUATIONS BIAS

Simultaneous equations bias can occur when an independent variable is correlated with the error term of the relationship being estimated. Our primary interest is in the impact of medical care on health (using mortality as a health indicator). However, the theory developed in chapter 2 clearly showed that the quantity of medical care consumed depends on the level of health desired and the initial stock of health. Very simply, sick people generally consume more medical care than well people. If the medical care variables are in fact correlated with the error term of the production function, then their parameter estimates will be both biased and inconsistent.[6]

Since all of the theory's equations have not been specified, we shall use the method of instrumental variables (IV) to obtain unbiased parameter estimates of the medical care variables. The instruments will be obtained by regressing each medical care variable against exogenous variables from each part of the overall theory.

4. SPECIFICATION BIAS

Specification bias refers to the problem of omitting key variables from the production function. The bias resulting from omitted variables depends on the correlations between the omitted factor and both the dependent variable and the other independent variables. In this study, this problem is most likely to arise because of the difficulty of observing environmental or behavioral factors which may influence mortality rates. Air pollution, water pollution, and exposure to toxic elements are examples of the former. Cigarette smoking, exercise habits, and diet are examples of the latter.

Fortunately, these factors are not likely to be highly correlated with the measures of medical care. This assumption will be tested indirectly for the environmental variables by regressing the medical care variables against several measures of environmental conditions. A low R^2 will imply that the latter can be safely omitted.[7] No direct measures of personal behavior are available for this study. However, it seems unlikely that personal habits themselves will be highly correlated with medical care use. There may, of course, be an indirect link through the effect of personal behavior on health, but this is essentially the simultaneous equation problem.

Another aspect of specification bias is the inclusion of extraneous variables. This does not generally bias parameter estimates, but it can lead to higher estimated standard errors, and thus less reliable parameter estimates. This problem will be addressed by deleting variables which are consistently statistically insignificant in the preliminary regressions.

Preliminary Specification and Results

Chapters 4 and 5 described the mortality rates and medical care variables used in the analysis. Other potential variables include proxies for variations in medical care quality, environmental characteristics, health stock variables, and behavior/lifestyle variables. This section first describes these other independent variables and then reports the results of statistical tests of the methodological issues raised in the preceding section. The latter includes pooling cohorts, elimination of extraneous variables, choice of functional form, simultaneous equations bias, and testing for heteroskedasticity.

1. OTHER INDEPENDENT VARIABLES

a. Medical Care Quality Several variables will be used as potential controls for variations in medical care quality, physician productivity, and the composition of medical services. These include the proportion of physicians who are GPs, the presence of a medical school, the number of foreign medical school graduates currently in residency training (per capita), and the proportion of occupied hospital beds in hospitals with 11 or more services and facilities as defined by the American Hospital Association. A more indirect approach to controlling for quality variations focuses on the difference between *expected* outcomes for a cause of death category which should be amenable to medical treatment and the observed outcome. Following Silver, another quality control proxy is the difference between the actual and expected mortality rates from flu and pneumonia.[8]

b. Environmental Variables For variables measuring environmental characteristics, we attempt to focus on water quality, air quality, climate, and occupational hazards. Because these factors are unlikely to be closely associated with the consumption of medical care, the choice of specific measures was guided primarily by data availability. Water quality will be measured by two variables: the percentage of households which obtain water from public systems and the percentage of households with public sewer connections. Climate is also measured by two variables: mean January temperature and mean annual precipitation. Air quality will be approximated by an index of suspended particles in the air. Finally, exposure to occupational hazards will be measured by the proportion of cohort members in mining, construction, chemical, rubber, paper, and metal smelting industries. We expect a high index of suspended particles and a high proportion of workers in hazardous industries to be positively associated with mortality rates. We have no expectations about the signs of the other variables.

  c. *Health Stock Variables* The health stock variables group attempts to control for variations in cohorts' initial health stocks or health statuses. As noted in the theory section, variations in health stock affect not only the efficiency of health production but also the demand for and the marginal cost of health. However, since a direct health measure is not available, a set of proxy variables must be used.

  Three potentially major sources of variation in health stock are controlled for by stratifying the population into age, sex, and race cohorts. Within each cohort, the distribution of national origins will be measured by the proportions of people born in Latin American, Eastern European, and Asian and African countries, respectively, and the proportion of people of Spanish heritage or descent. These variables obviously do not identify the nature or strength of the relationship, if any, between genetics, heredity, national origin, and mortality. Since this is not an objective of this study, however, it is not essential that the causal links, if any, underlying these relationships be explicitly identified. Other variables measuring health stock reflect labor force participation, migration, fertility, disability, and veteran status.

  d. *Behavior/Life-Style Variables* The final set of variables in the model contains proxies for the effects of variations in life-style or behavior. It was pointed out earlier that there are no direct measures for small geographic areas of key aspects of health behavior such as diet, smoking, drinking, exercise, and rest. An indirect proxy for variations in alcohol consumption will be constructed by estimating the expected number of deaths from cirrhosis of the liver and alcoholism by cohort and area. The difference between the expected and actual death rate will be used as an index of the effects of alcohol consumption. A variable representing cigarette consumption will be constructed from state data on cigarette sales per capita. We will attempt to control for other behavioral differences using measures of income, education, occupation, and marital status. All have been significantly associated with mortality rates in previous studies. Education also plays a potentially significant role in the model as a factor affecting the efficiency of health production.

  e. *Other Exogenous Variables* The model's remaining variables are drawn from other parts of the overall theory of health and medical care. Although these variables do not enter the health production function directly, they will be used to generate instrumental variables for the medical care measures. The set of other exogenous variables includes population density, percentages of the county group's population living on farms and in urban areas, the net migration rate of the county group's population, and nursing home beds per capita. In general, these variables may be thought of as factors affecting the supply of medical care resources in an area.

Table A.1 summarizes all of the health production function's independent variables and indicates their data sources and expected signs. (Exogenous variables from other parts of the model are not included.)

2. POOLING AND DELETION OF EXTRANEOUS VARIABLES

Only a single mortality rate, deaths from all causes per 1,000 cohort members, will be used in this phase of the analysis. All regressions reported are based on analysis of age-sex-race-specific cohorts with at least 750 people. Since the data from the 1970 Census represent a 2 percent sample of the population in each cohort, this implies that the personal characteristics' measures are based on samples of at least 15 people in a cohort. Cells with fewer than 15 sample individuals were deleted from further study on the grounds that the resulting estimates of the cohort's characteristics would not be sufficiently reliable for analysis. All of the white cohorts satisfied this constraint. However, only 57 percent of the under-age-65 black cohorts and 38 percent of the 65-and-older black cohorts met the minimum sample requirements. Therefore, adjoining age-specific black cohorts were pooled to form cohorts spanning the ages 45 to 64 and 65 and older. Pooling cohorts in this way provided samples ranging in size from 294 to 428 county groups for estimating the mortality production functions for blacks.

A similar pooling strategy was also explored for the white cohorts. Regressions were first estimated separately for each 10-year-age cohort, and then for pooled pairs of 10-year-age cohorts. The second set of equations combined observations for 45-to-54 and 55-to-64 age groups, and the 65-to-74 and 75-and-older age groups. Pooling in this fashion essentially doubles the number of observations in each regression, thus increasing the power of the statistical tests. Examination of the parameters of key variables (education, income, physician stock, and Medicare expenditures) indicated that the coefficients for the pooled regressions were approximately averages of the coefficients of the individual cohorts. Although not formally tested, the values seem sufficiently close to permit pooling. This procedure greatly simplifies the exposition and reporting of results.

The next phase of the preliminary analysis investigated the specification of the estimating equation, focusing on high simple correlations among

TABLE A.1
DEFINITIONS OF INDEPENDENT VARIABLES

VARIABLE	DEFINITION	EXPECTED SIGN	SOURCE
1. Medical Care Variables			
MDPOP	Active, nonfederal patient care physicians per 1,000 population	−	1
NURSPOP	Employed hospital and nonhospital registered and licensed practical nurses per 1,000 population	−	1
BEDPOP	Occupied nonfederal, short-term, general hospital beds per 1,000 population	−	1
MDSR[a]	Active, nonfederal patient care physicians per 1,000 cohort members	−	1
NURSR[a]	Employed hospital and nonhospital registered and licensed practical nurses per 1,000 cohort members	−	1
BEDR[a]	Occupied nonfederal, short-term, general hospital beds per 1,000 cohort members	−	1
MDCREXP	Total Medicare expenditures per enrollee	−	1
PGP	Percentage of general practitioners	?	1
LGBEDS	Percentage of beds in hospitals with 11 or more services	?	1
MEDSCH	Equals 1 if a medical school is present, 0 otherwise	−	1
FORPC	Graduates of foreign medical schools in residency training, per capita	?	1
EXFLU[b]	Excess deaths from flu and pneumonia, by cohort	+	2
2. Environmental Variables			
PWS	Percentage of households with water from public systems	?	3
PSC	Percentage of households with public sewer connections	?	3
MJT	Mean January temperature	?	4
RAIN	Annual precipitation	?	4
SUN	Mean annual percentage sunshine	?	4
PARTS	Index of suspended particles	+	5
HIND	Proportion of workers in hazardous industries (construction, mining, smelting and refining, paper, rubber and chemicals), by cohort	+	3

TABLE A.1 (cont'd)
DEFINITIONS OF INDEPENDENT VARIABLES

Variable	Definition	Expected Sign	Source
3. Health Stock Variables			
AVA	Average age	+	3
EEUR	Percentage born in Eastern European countries, by cohort	?	3
LATIN	Percentage born in Latin American countries, by cohort	?	3
ASAFR	Percentage born in Asian or African countries, by cohort	?	3
USB	Percentage born in the U.S., by cohort	?	3
DISABL	Percentage with work- or activity-limiting disabilities, under age 65 cohorts only	+	3
NILF	Percentage not in labor force, female cohorts	+	3
WORK68	Percentage last worked after 1968, male cohorts	−	3
SPAN	Percentage Spanish heritage or descent, by cohort	?	3
VET	Percentage veterans, male cohorts	?	3
KIDS	Average number of children ever born, female cohorts	?	3
MIGR	Percentage who resided in different state five years earlier, by cohort	−	3
4. Behavior/Life Style			
AHG	Average highest grade of school completed, by cohort	−	3
TFI	Average family income, by cohort	−	3
EI	Average earned income (wages, salaries, professional, and farm income), by cohort	−	3
UI	Average unearned income (TFI-EI), by cohort	−	3
CIGS	Cigarettes sold per capita in the state	+	6
MAR	Percentage married, by cohort	−	3
WID	Percentage widowed, by cohort	+	3
DS	Percentage divorced or separated, by cohort	+	3
NM	Percentage never married, by cohort	+	3
AGEMAR	Average age at first marriage, by cohort	?	3

TABLE A.1 (cont'd)
DEFINITIONS OF INDEPENDENT VARIABLES

VARIABLE	DEFINITION	EXPECTED SIGN	SOURCE
PROF	Percentage in professional, technical, and other white-collar occupations, by cohort	?	3
FARM	Percentage in farm occupations, by cohort	?	3
EXALCIR[b]	Excess deaths from cirrhosis of the liver and alcoholism, by cohort	+	2

SOURCES: 1. Area Resource File.
2. NCHS Mortality File.
3. Two percent sample, 1970 Census of Population.
4. *County and City Data Book, 1972.*
5. EPA, *Air Quality Data-1970 Annual Statistics.*
6. *Tobacco Tax Council, The Tax Burden on Tobacco, 1977.*
a. See Jack Hadley, "Does Medical Care Affect Health?" Appendix 3 contains details on construction of these variables.
b. The difference between actual and predicted deaths for each cohort and county group.

variables (a possible source of multicollinearity) and the elimination of extraneous variables. Variables were eliminated if they consistently had t-statistics less than 1. This process suggested several ways in which the final specification could be made more parsimonious.

First, two sets of variables measuring marital status and national origin were collapsed into single variables. Widowed, divorced, separated, and never married are measured by their complement, percentage married. Similarly, the distribution of each cohort by national origin will be represented by its complement, percentage U.S. born. Second, high correlations were observed between occupation (professional, farmer) and income and industry (agriculture). Therefore, the occupation variables were deleted. Third, several of the medical care stock variables and the quality/service mix proxies exhibited high correlations. This was particularly true for the measures of employed nurses and occupied hospital beds, which usually had correlation coefficients larger than 0.9. This suggests that these two resources are distributed in essentially fixed proportions, and that one of them can be deleted without serious loss of information. As will be shown next, including more than one medical care resource variable generally resulted in highly unstable parameter estimates.

Of the quality/service mix proxies, the presence of a medical school and the proportion of occupied hospital beds in large hospitals were almost always insignificant. The percentage of physicians who are general practitioners and the number of foreign-trained residents per capita were also highly correlated with the supply of physicians. These two variables generally had the expected positive signs and were occasionally significant in the regressions for whites. However, the coefficient of the medical care variable seemed to be sensitive to their inclusion. Therefore, all four of these variables were excluded.

Finally, the set of proxy variables measuring environmental characteristics had little systematic effect on the dependent variables. In addition, these variables had a very low association with physician supply. (Regressions of the physician stock against the environmental variables produced R^2s of about 0.15). Several of these variables are subject to a high rate of missing values, and therefore have an adverse impact on the number of cases available for analysis. Thus, they were deleted from the final specifications of the equations reported in the next subsection and in chapter 5. The impact of these variables will be considered in a separate phase of the analysis.

3. CHOICES OF FUNCTIONAL FORM, MEDICAL CARE MEASURE, AND ESTIMATION METHOD

What is the proper mathematical form of the production function, and how should medical care use be measured? Two functional forms are examined. Letting Y = the mortality rate, X = vector of medical care variables, and Z = vector of all other variables, the two forms can be represented by

$$y = a + \alpha x + \delta Z \tag{A.9}$$

$$y = a' + \alpha' x + \beta X + \delta' Z, \tag{A.10}$$

where lower case y and x represent logarithmic values.

In general, we expect that $\alpha < 0$ and $\beta > 0$, that is, increased use of medical care reduces mortality rates up to a point. After that point, however, more medical care may have no further impact on mortality rates and could conceivably increase mortality rates through iatrogenic factors. If $\beta = 0$, then the second form reduces to the first.

Three approaches to measuring medical care were examined: (1) stocks of physicians, nurses, and hospital beds per 1,000 people in the county group; (2) cohort-specific stocks of physicians, nurses, and hospital beds per 1,000 cohort members;[9] and (3) Medicare expenditures per enrollee. In each of the first two approaches, the physician variable includes only active, nonfederal, patient care physicians, the nurse variable consists of employed registered and licensed practical nurses, and the beds variable of occupied beds in short-term community hospitals.

Equations (A.9) and (A.10) were estimated by ordinary least squares for each of the three sets of medical care variables. For the first two sets, the equations were also estimated with the physician variable as the only medical care proxy. Thus, four equations were estimated for each of the two stocks-of-resources approaches to measuring medical care.

Table A.2 reports the estimated coefficients of the various medical care variables for the eight pooled cohorts. Consider first equations 1 and 2 of specification set 1. These equations use physicians per 1,000 population as the medical care measure. Only one of the eight equation 1 estimates (white females, 65 and older) has both the anticipated sign and is significantly different from zero, and none of the equation 2 estimates meet the sign and statistical significance criteria. In the only two cohorts with a significant medical care effect (white females, 45 to 64, and black males, 45 to 64), the signs are the opposite of those expected.

Coefficient estimates of the cohort-specific physician variables (specification set 2) attain statistical significance more often than in set 1, but have the incorrect signs in three of the eight cohorts. The equation 2 estimates have the correct sign and attain statistical significance only for one cohort (black males, 65 and older).

Adding the measures of nurses and occupied hospital beds, equations 3 and 4, clearly increases the extent of multicollinearity. In no case do all variables have the expected signs. Although individual coefficients attain statistical significance, the pattern of magnitudes and sign changes, particularly in comparing equations 3 and 4, indicates the sensitivity of the estimates to the variables included. (Correlation coefficients between physicians and nurses per 1,000 population were between 0.64 and 0.74, and between cohort-specific nurses and beds about 0.9).

Turning to specification set 3, which uses Medicare expenditures per enrollee as the proxy for medical care use, all equation 1 estimates have the correct sign and all but one are also statistically significant. The equation 2 estimates appear much less plausible. Only one of the βs is significantly different from zero, and it has the incorrect sign (white females, 45 to 64).

Overall, these results strongly suggest that the simple Cobb-Douglas production function with medical care measured as the natural logarithm of Medicare expenditures per enrollee is the best form to use. As noted in chapter 4, there are several factors which a priori reinforce the empirical results. Subsequent analyses and results will therefore be based on this combinaton of functional form and medical care measure.

Given the selection of Medicare expenditures per enrollee (MCDREXP) as the measure of medical care use, the next issue investigated was the choice of an estimation method. As noted, there is reason to believe that medical care use is correlated with the error term of the health production function. This can be easily shown by equations (A.11) and (A.12), where Y = mortality rate, X = medical care use, ϵ and ξ are the error terms of the two equations, and α, β, γ, and δ are the parameters to be estimated. All other variables are omitted for convenience.

$$Y = \alpha + \beta X + \epsilon, \; \beta < 0 \text{ (health production)} \tag{A.11}$$

$$X = \gamma + \delta Y + \xi, \; \delta > 0 \text{ (demand for medical care)} \tag{A.12}$$

Solving these two equations for Y and X shows clearly that X depends on ϵ, the error term of the health production function.

$$Y = \frac{\alpha + \beta \gamma}{1 - \beta \delta} + \frac{\beta \xi + \epsilon}{1 - \beta \delta} \tag{A.13}$$

$$X = \gamma + \frac{\delta(\alpha + \beta \gamma)}{1 - \beta \delta} + \frac{\delta(\beta \xi + \epsilon)}{1 - \beta \delta} + \xi \tag{A.14}$$

This suggests that a simultaneous-equations estimation method, in this case the instrumental variables (IV) method, is preferable to the use of ordinary least squares (OLS). Inappropriate application of OLS will in general result in parameter estimates which are both biased and inconsistent. The direction of the bias can be assessed by evaluating the OLS expression for $\hat{\beta}$,

$$\hat{\beta} = (X'X)^{-1}X'Y = (X'X)^{-1}X'\beta X + (X'X)^{-1}X'\epsilon \tag{A.15}$$

$$= \beta + (X'X)^{-1}X'\epsilon$$

Since $(X'X)^{-1}$ is a constant, the expected value of $\hat{\beta}$ depends on the covariance of $X'\epsilon$.

$$\text{Cov}(X'\epsilon) = E[X - E(X)]E[\epsilon - E(\epsilon)] \tag{A.16}$$

$$= E[X'\epsilon] - E[X] \cdot E[\epsilon].$$

Since $E[\epsilon] = 0$, the second term drops out, leaving

$$\text{Cov}(X'\epsilon) = \frac{\delta}{1 - \beta \delta}\sigma^2 + \frac{1}{1 - \beta \delta}\sigma_{\xi\epsilon}. \tag{A.17}$$

This expression will be positive if $\sigma_{\xi\epsilon} < 0$.

TABLE A.2
COEFFICIENTS OF MEDICAL CARE VARIABLES, PRELIMINARY ANALYSES
(male cohorts)

	WHITE MALES, 45–64				BLACK MALES, 45–64			
	1	2	3	4	1	2	3	4
Specification-Set 1 (OLS)								
Log MDs per 1000 pop.	.012	.004	−.011	.034	.067*	.104**	.068**	.076
MDs per 1000 pop.		.006		−.045**		−.028		.003
Log beds per 1000 pop.			.034*	.021			.018	−.047
Beds per 1000 pop.				.006				.013
Log nurses per 1000 pop.			.013	−.279*			−.018	.287
Nurses per 1000 pop.				.061*				−.069
Specification-Set 2 (OLS)								
Log MDs per 1000 cohort	.063*	.073*	.029	.049**	.029**	.063**	.042*	.071*
MDs per 1000 cohort		−.005		−.009		−.012**		−.009**
Log beds per 1000 cohort			.041**	.017			−.010	.006
Beds per 1000 cohort				.004				−.001
Log nurses per 1000 cohort			.022	.045			−.008	.006
Nurses per 1000 cohort				−.006				−.004
Specification-Set 3 (OLS)								
Log Medicare expenditures per enrollee	−.098*	−.085			−.067	.131		
Medicare expenditures per enrollee		NS				−.001		
Specification-Set 3 (IV)								
Log Medicare expenditures per enrollee	−.317*	−.460*			.043	−.457		
Medicare expenditures per enrollee		NS				.002		

TABLE A.2 (cont'd)
(male cohorts)

	WHITE MALES, 65+				BLACK MALES, 65+			
	1	2	3	4	1	2	3	4
Specification-Set 1 *(OLS)*								
Log MDs per 1000 pop.	-.006	-.025	-.006	.015	.009	-.028	.021	-.024
MDs per 1000 pop.		.015		-.019		.029		.040
Log beds per 1000 pop.			.014	-.053**			.049	.072
Beds per 1000 pop.				.017*				-.007
Log nurses per 1000 pop.			-.018	-.089			-.070	.043
Nurses per 1000 pop.				.015				-.024
Specification-Set 2 *(OLS)*								
Log MDs per 1000 cohort	.036*	.057*	.025*	.050*	-.009	-.039*	-.026*	-.051**
MDs per 1000 cohort		-.007		-.008		.007*		.006
Log beds per 1000 cohort			.023	-.042			-.014	-.008
Beds per 1000 cohort				.005*				-.001
Log nurses per 1000 cohort			-.002	.062			.042	.034
Nurses per 1000 cohort				-.009**				.002
Specification-Set 3 *(OLS)*								
Log Medicare expenditures per enrollee	-.051*	-.051**			-.165*	.084		
Medicare expenditures per enrollee		NS				-.001		
Specification-Set 3 *(IV)*								
Log Medicare expenditures per enrollee	-.123*	-.457*			-.166*	.675*		
Medicare expenditures per enrollee		.001*				.002**		

*Significant at 99 percent confidence level.
**Significant at 95 percent confidence level.
NS Less than .0005.

TABLE A.2 (cont'd)
(female cohorts)

	WHITE FEMALES, 45-64				BLACK FEMALES, 45-64			
	1	2	3	4	1	2	3	4
Specification-Set 1 *(OLS)*								
Log MDs per 1000 pop.	-.020	.060*	-.037*	.046	-.020	-.011	-.070*	-.095
MDs per 1000 pop.		-.066*		-.069*		-.007		.025
Log beds per 1000 pop.			-.014	.019			.035	.031
Beds per 1000 pop.				-.005				NS
Log nurses per 1000 pop.			.061*	-.083			.078	.271
Nurses per 1000 pop.				.027				-.043
Specification-Set 2 *(OLS)*								
Log MDs per 1000 cohort	-.007	.095*	-.027**	.087*	-.048*	-.015	-.099*	-.069*
MDs per 1000 cohort		-.038*		-.045*		-.007**		-.006
Log beds per 1000 cohort			-.056*	-.005			.078	.110**
Beds per 1000 cohort				-.008				-.003
Log nurses per 1000 cohort			.082*	.009			-.024	-.053
Nurses per 1000 cohort				.021				.004
Specification-Set 3 *(OLS)*								
Log Medicare expenditures per enrollee	-.056*	.372*			-.149**	.229		
Medicare expenditures per enrollee		-.001*				-.001		
Specification-Set 3 *(IV)*								
Log Medicare expenditures per enrollee	-.126*	.726*			-.108	-.108		
Medicare expenditures per enrollee		-.003*				NS		

TABLE A.2 (cont'd)
(female cohorts)

	WHITE FEMALES, 65+				BLACK FEMALES, 65+			
	1	2	3	4	1	2	3	4
Specification-Set 1 (OLS)								
Log MDs per 1000 pop.	−.028*	.008	−.034*	−.010	−.037	−.086	.009	−.041
MDs per 1000 pop.		−.023		−.019		.039		.040
Log beds per 1000 pop.			−.007	.005			.040	−.039
Beds per 1000 pop.				−.002				.016
Log nurses per 1000 pop.			.025	NS			−.131**	.088
Nurses per 1000 pop.				.004				−.048
Specification-Set 2 (OLS)								
Log MDs per 1000 cohort	−.010	.052*	−.015	.051*	−.052*	−.023	−.041**	−.013
MDs per 1000 cohort		−.019*		−.021*		−.008		−.007
Log beds per 1000 cohort			−.011	−.043			−.016	−.094
Beds per 1000 cohort				.003				.009
Log nurses per 1000 cohort			.019	.054			NS	.058
Nurses per 1000 cohort				−.005				−.012
Specification-Set 3 (OLS)								
Log Medicare expenditures per enrollee	−.079*	−.042			−.169*	−.063		
Medicare expenditures per enrollee		NS				NS		
Specification-Set 3 (IV)								
Log Medicare expenditures per enrollee	−.141*	−.186			−.183*	−.904*		
Medicare expenditures per enrollee		NS				.002**		

*Significant at 99 percent confidence level.
**Significant at 95 percent confidence level.
NS Less than .0005.

In general, it seems safe to assume that the last condition holds as specified. Random events which increase mortality rates, such as epidemics or natural disasters, will also increase the use of medical care. At the same time, unspecified factors which influence medical care use, for example, attitudes or perceptions about medical care, are unlikely to have any effect on mortality rates or health status. Under these conditions the OLS estimate of β will have a positive bias, that is, toward zero.

Table A.3 reports both the OLS and IV estimates (from table A.2) of the coefficient of the log of Medicare expenditures per enrollee. For each of the white cohorts the IV estimate is larger (in absolute value) than the OLS estimate. The difference is approximately twofold except for white males, 45 to 64, for whom the IV estimate is almost four times larger. These results imply that the particular instruments used in the IV estimation are appropriate for the white cohorts.

The results for the black cohorts are less clearcut, however. The OLS and IV estimates are nearly identical for the two elderly cohorts. For the middle-aged cohorts, the IV estimates are smaller than the OLS estimates and one has an implausibly positive, though statistically insignificant sign.

A possible explanation of the apparent superiority of the OLS estimates for the black cohorts is that Medicare expenditures per enrollee may itself be an acceptable instrumental variable for the unobserved measure of medical care expenditures per capita in the black cohorts. This would be the case if Medicare expenditures per enrollee, whose value is determined

TABLE A.3

ORDINARY LEAST SQUARES AND INSTRUMENTAL VARIABLES ESTIMATES
OF MDCREXP's COEFFICIENT, DEATHS FROM ALL CAUSES, BY COHORT

	COEFFICIENT	
COHORT	ORDINARY LEAST SQUARES	INSTRUMENTAL VARIABLES
White males, 45–64	−.098*	−.317*
White males, 65+	−.051*	−.123*
White females, 45–64	−.056*	−.126*
White females, 65+	−.079*	−.141*
Black males, 45–64	−.067	.043
Black males, 65+	−.165*	−.166*
Black females, 45–64	−.149*	−.108
Black females, 65+	−.169*	−.183*

*Statistically significant at 95 percent confidence level or higher.

primarily by the behavior of whites, is correlated with blacks' medical care expenditures but not with random events which influence blacks' mortality rates. In effect, this variable is already an acceptable instrument for the unobserved, medical care expenditures per capita for blacks.

The final estimation issue explored was heteroskedasticity of the error term. Following Johnston, the null hypothesis of homoskedasticity can be tested by ordering county groups by population, dividing the sample into three partitions, and estimating the health production functions separately for each of the two extreme partitions.[10] The ratio of the sums of squared residuals has an F-distribution. Since the alternative hypothesis is that the variance decreases as county group population increases, the null hypothesis is rejected if F is smaller than the appropriate critical value.

The calculated ratios using both ordinary and instrumental variables estimation methods ranged in value from 0.34 to 0.71, with eight larger than 0.54. Since the sample sizes are relatively large for each cohort, the appropriate critical value of F at the 95 percent confidence level is approximately 0.8. Since all the ratios are less than 0.8, this indicates that the data are inconsistent with the assumption of a homoskedastic error term. Visual inspection of the scatter of residuals plotted against population suggested that the degree of heteroskedasticity was small, however. Therefore, no adjustments were made to the data in order to reduce computational burden.

APPENDIX B

COUNTIES WITH LARGE VALUES OF TWO RANKING CRITERIA, SELECTED STATES

LEGEND FOR MAPS B.1 THROUGH B.8

⦿ Places of 100,000 or more inhabitants
● Places of 50,000 to 100,000 inhabitants
☐ Central cities of SMSAs with fewer than
   50,000 inhabitants
○ Places of 25,000 to 50,000 inhabitants
   outside SMSAs

 Standard Metropolitan Statistical Areas (SMSAs)

Among 500 counties with the largest values of
population per patient care physician

Among 500 counties with largest values of
deaths averted per $100,000 increase in
medical care spending

MAP B.1

COUNTIES WITH LARGE VALUES OF TWO RANKING CRITERIA,
ARKANSAS, 1970

See legend on page 203.

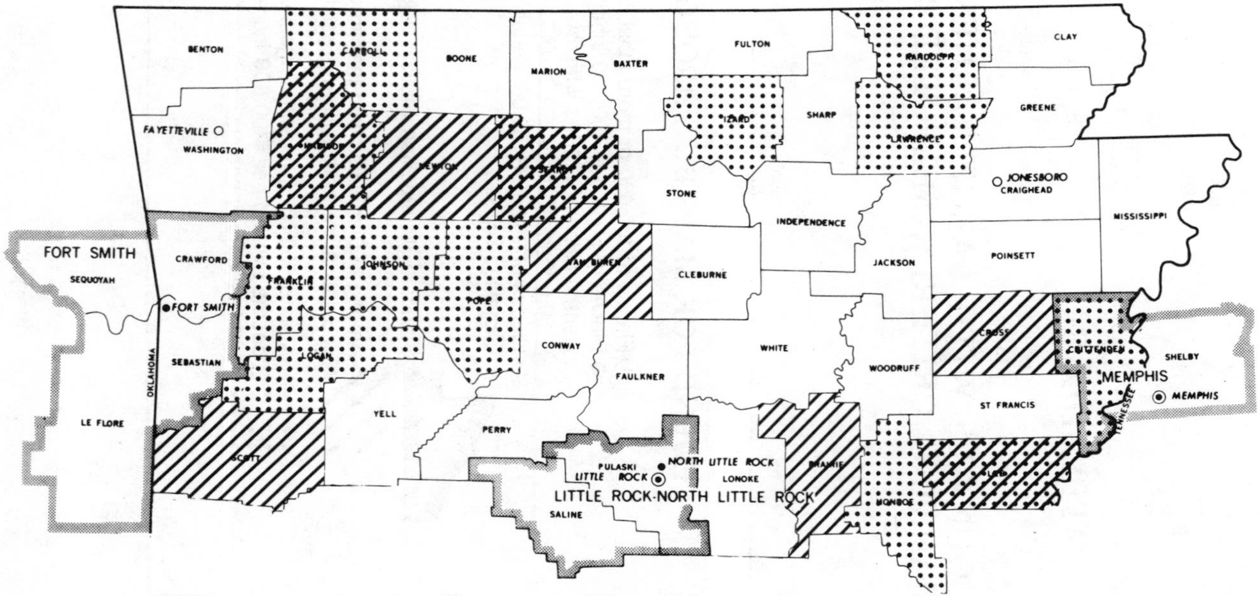

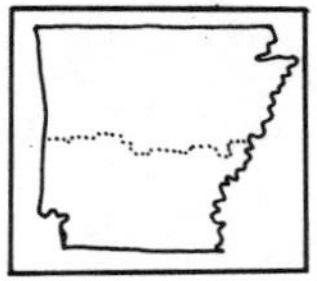

MAP B.1 (cont'd)

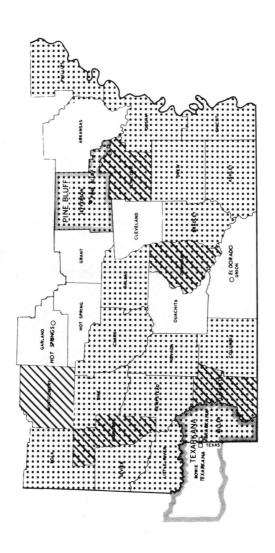

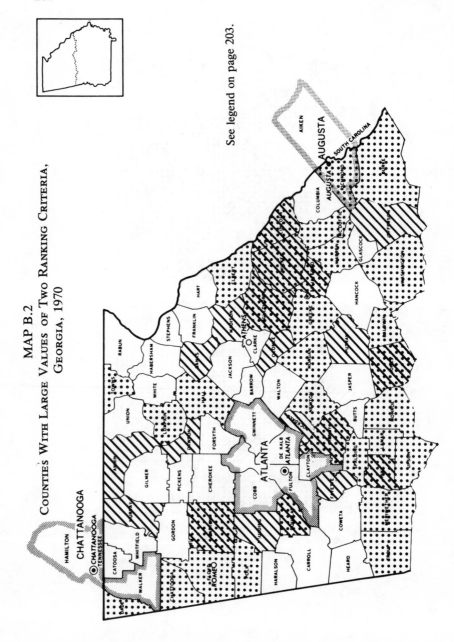

MAP B.2

COUNTIES WITH LARGE VALUES OF TWO RANKING CRITERIA,
GEORGIA, 1970

See legend on page 203.

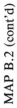

MAP B.2 (cont'd)

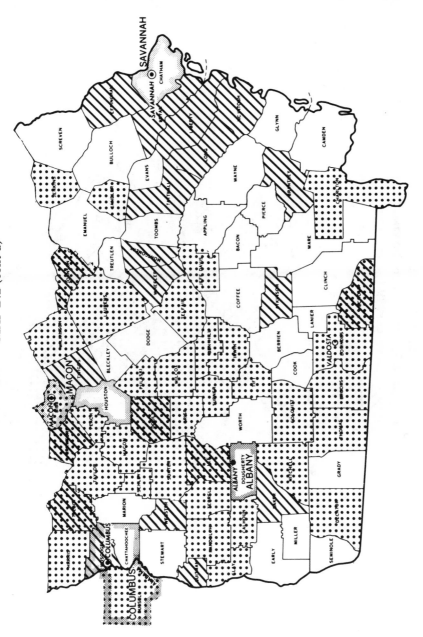

MAP B.3
COUNTIES WITH LARGE VALUES OF TWO RANKING CRITERIA
KENTUCKY, 1970

See legend on page 203.

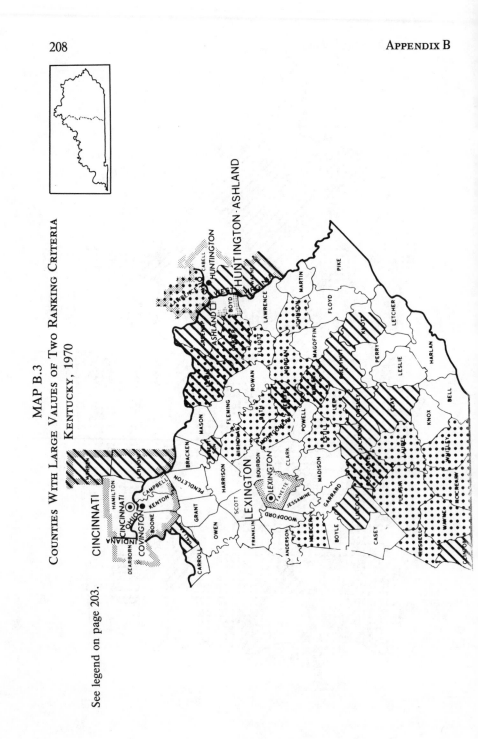

MAP B.3 (cont'd)

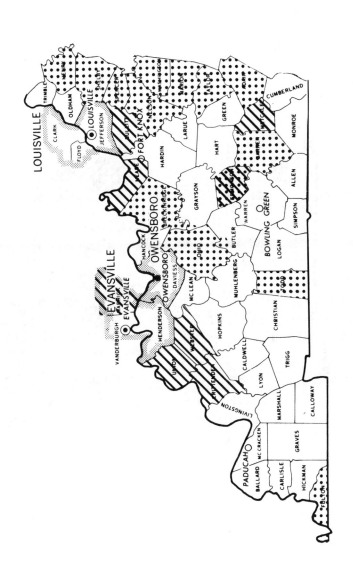

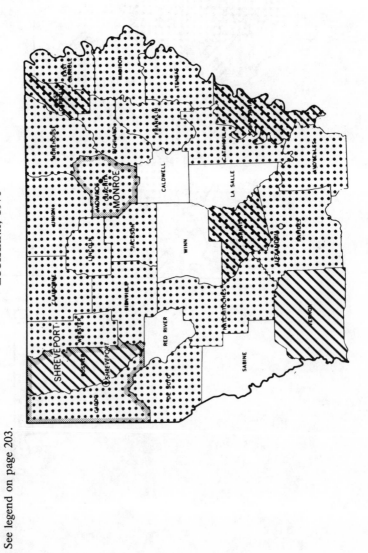

MAP B.4
COUNTIES WITH LARGE VALUES OF TWO RANKING CRITERIA,
LOUISIANA, 1970

See legend on page 203.

MAP B.4 (cont'd)

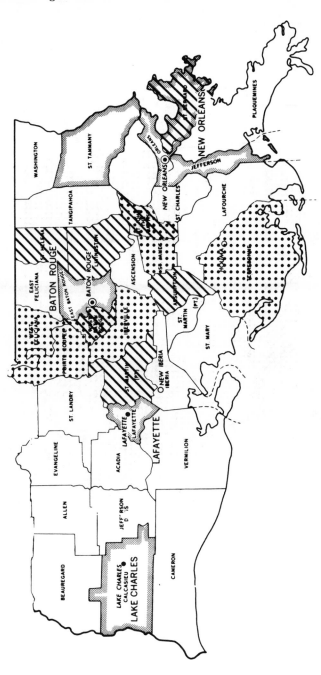

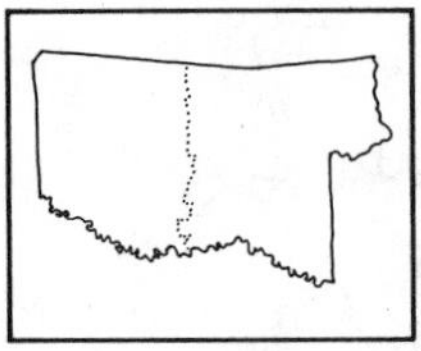

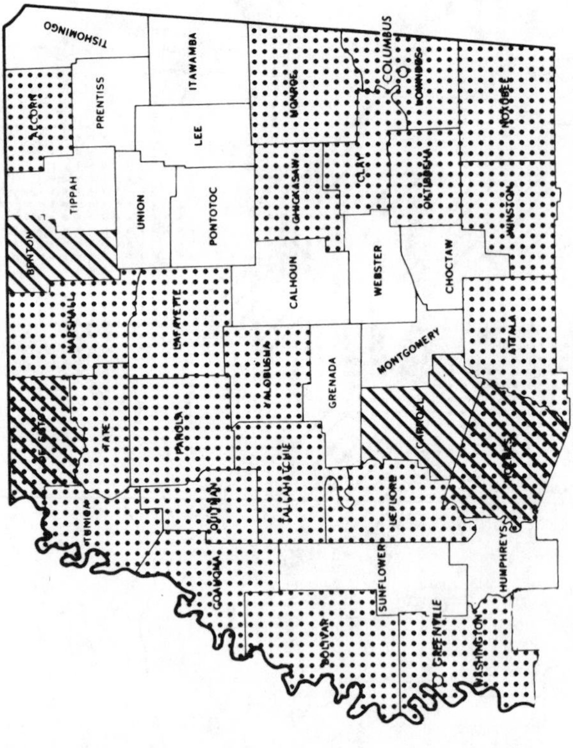

MAP B.5
COUNTIES WITH LARGE VALUES OF TWO RANKING CRITERIA,
MISSISSIPPI, 1970

See legend on page 203.

MAP B.5 (cont'd)

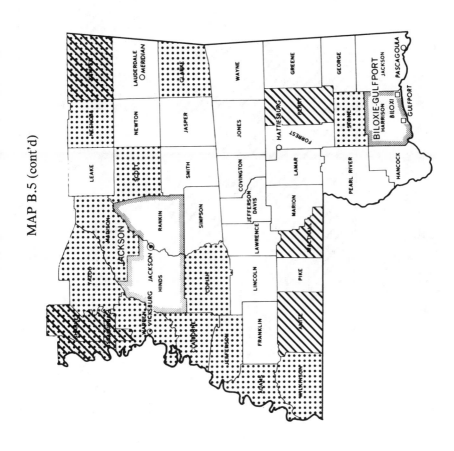

MAP B.6

COUNTIES WITH LARGE VALUES OF TWO RANKING CRITERIA,
MISSOURI, 1970

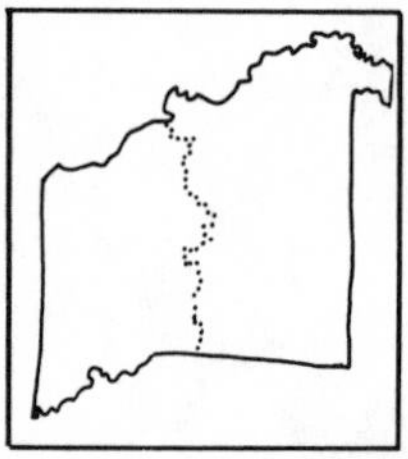

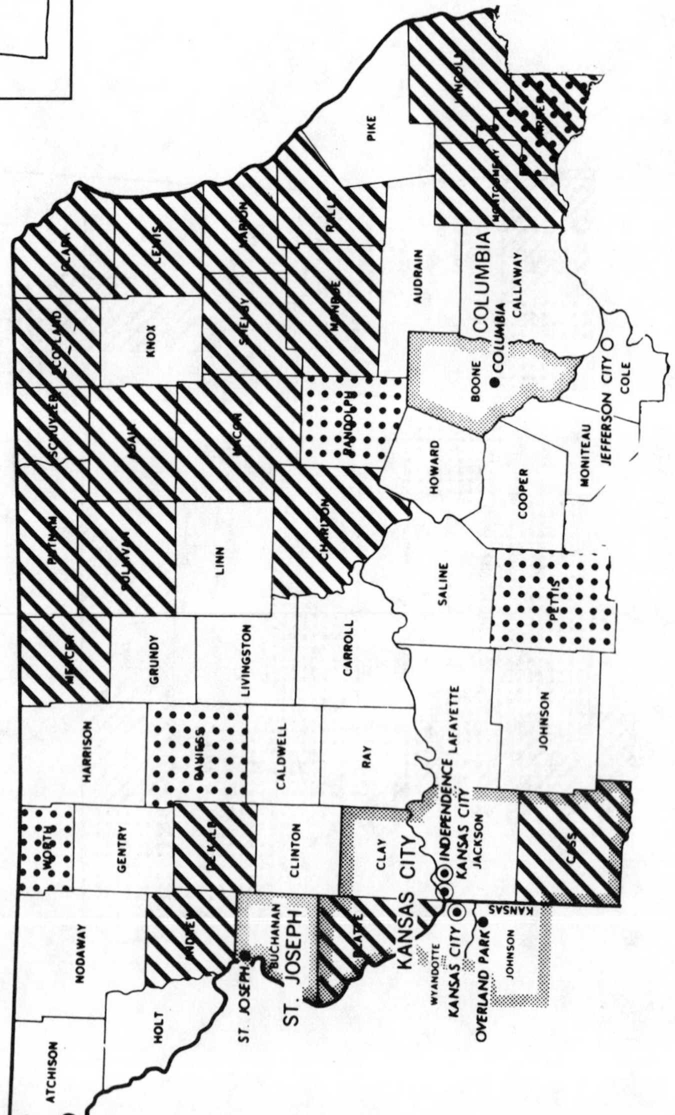

See legend on page 203.

MAP B.6 (cont'd)

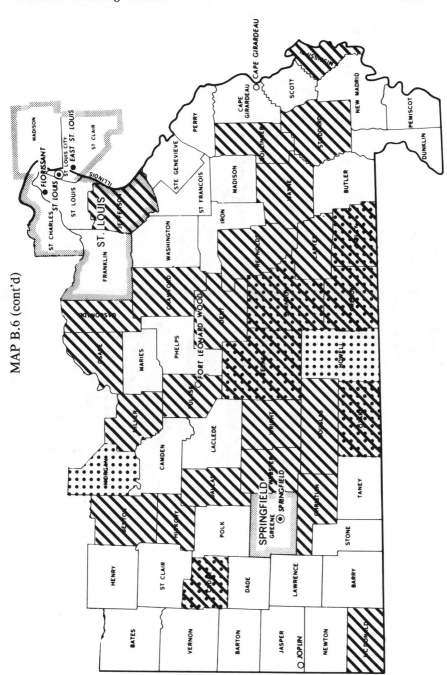

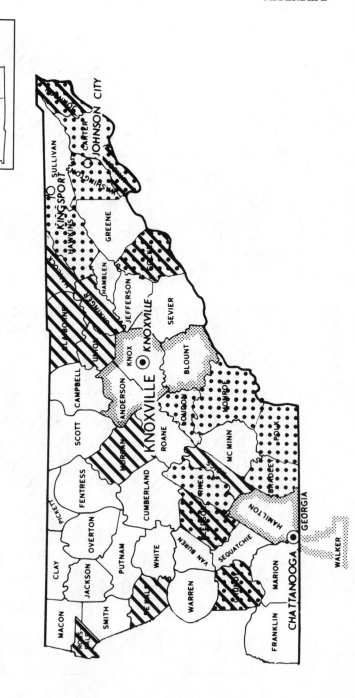

MAP B.7

COUNTIES WITH LARGE VALUES OF TWO RANKING CRITERIA,
TENNESSEE, 1970

See legend on page 203.

MAP B.7 (cont'd)

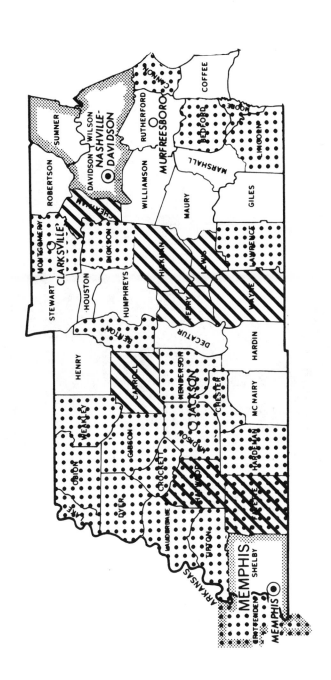

MAP B.8

COUNTIES WITH LARGE VALUES OF TWO RANKING CRITERIA,
VIRGINIA, 1970

See legend on page 203.

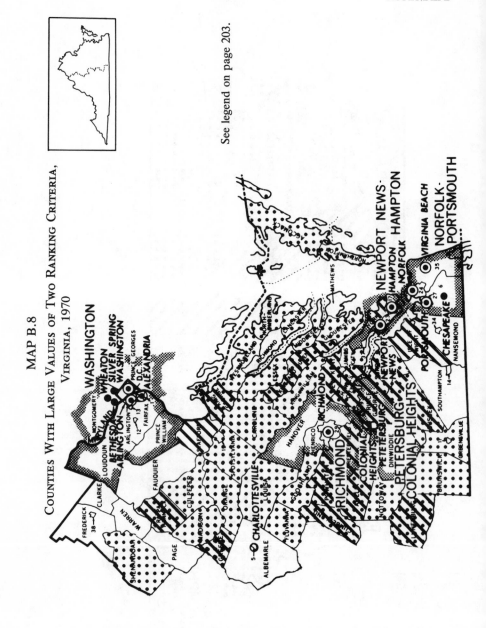

MAP B.8 (cont'd)

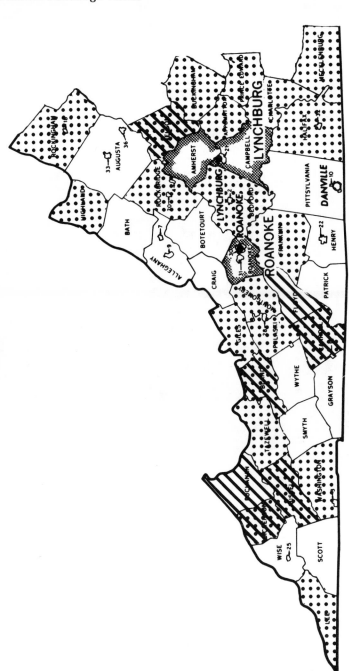

NOTES

NOTES TO CHAPTER 1

1. See, for example, Victor Fuchs, "The Contribution of Health Services to the American Economy," in *Essays in the Economics of Health and Medical Care*, ed. Victor Fuchs (New York: National Bureau of Economic Research, 1972), pp. 15-30; Aviva Berk, Lynn Paringer, and Selma Mushkin, "The Economic Cost of Illness—Fiscal 1975," *Medical Care* (September 1978): 785; Michael Grossman and Lee Benham, "Health, Hours, and Wages," (unpublished paper), National Bureau of Economic Research, March 1973, p. 39; and "National Health Expenditures and Related Measures," *Health Care Financing Trends* 1 (Fall 1979): 3.

2. "Summary of HEW Health Planning Goals," *The Blue Sheet*, supplement 22 (October 31, 1979): S-17, 18.

3. As of 1975, averages for these criteria were 16.41 deaths per 1,000 live births, 5.72 deaths per 1,000 people between the ages of 25 and 64, and 38.8 days of restricted activity per person aged 65 or older. Data are from U.S. Department of Health and Human Services, National Center for Health Statistics, "Final Mortality Statistics, 1978," *Monthly Vital Statistics Report* 29 (September 17, 1980): 16-17; and U.S. Department of Health, Education and Welfare, National Center for Health Statistics, *State Estimates of Disability and Utilization of Medical Services: United States, 1974-76* (Hyattsville, Md.: National Center for Health Statistics), p. 7.

4. Victor Fuchs, "Economics, Health, and Post-Industrial Society," *Milbank Memorial Fund Quarterly* 57 (Spring 1979): 155. See also, for example, Nathan Glazer, "Paradoxes of Health Care," *The Public Interest* 22 (Winter 1971): 62-77; John B. McKinlay and Sonja M. McKinlay, "The Questionable Contribution of Medical Measures to the Decline of Mortality in the United States in the Twentieth Century," *Health and Society* 55 (Summer 1977): 725; Victor Fuchs, *Who Shall Live?* (New York: Basic Books, 1974), p. 54; and Ivan Illich, *Medical Nemesis* (New York: Pantheon Books, 1976), pp. 15-26.

5. Robert M. Gibson and Marjorie S. Mueller, "National Health Expenditures, Fiscal Year 1976," *Social Security Bulletin* 40 (April 1977): 4.

6. See, for example, Illich, *Medical Nemesis*, pp. 26-32.

7. See, for example, Victor Fuchs and Marcia J. Kramer, *Determinants of Expenditures for Physicians' Services in The United States 1948-1968* (Rockville, Md.: U.S. Department of Health, Education and Welfare, 1972), p. 39; Lee Benham and Alexandra Benham, "The Impact of Incremental Medical Services on Health Status, 1963-1970," in *Equity in Health Services*, eds., Ronald Andersen, Joanna Kravits, and Odin W. Anderson (Cambridge, Mass.: Ballinger, 1975), p. 227; and Joseph Newhouse and Lindy J. Friedlander, "The Relationship Between Medical Resources and Measures of Health: Some Additional Evidence," *Journal of Human Resources* 15 (Spring 1980): 216.

8. Richard Auster, Irving Leveson, and Deborah Sarachek, "The Production of Health, An Exploratory Study," *Journal of Human Resources* 4 (Fall 1969): 430; Ronald L. Williams, "Explaining A Health Care Paradox," *Policy Sciences* 6 (March 1975): 91; and

David M. Kessner et al., *Infant Death: An Analysis by Maternal Risk and Health Care*, vol. 1 (Washington, D.C.: National Academy of Sciences, 1973), p. 1.

9. Fuchs, "Economics, Health, and Post-Industrial Society," p. 157. Also, see Fuchs, *Who Shall Live?*, p. 54.

10. U.S. Department of Health, Education and Welfare, "Health Manpower Shortages Areas: Criteria for Designation," *Federal Register* 43 (January 10, 1978): p. 1588.

11. Jack Hadley, "Alternative Methods of Evaluating Health Manpower Distribution," *Medical Care* 17 (October 1979): 1056.

12. Ibid., p. 1058.

13. Michael Grossman, *The Demand for Health* (New York: National Bureau of Economic Research, 1972).

NOTES TO CHAPTER 2

1. See, for example, Henrik L. Blum, *Planning for Health* (New York: Human Sciences Press), pp. 2-3; Lester B. Lave and Eugene P. Seskin, *Air Pollution and Human Health* (Baltimore: Johns Hopkins University Press, 1977), pp. 9-11.

2. Grossman, *The Demand for Health*.

3. Blum, *Planning for Health*, pp. 94-95.

4. Jan Kmenta, *Elements of Econometrics* (New York: Macmillan Publishing Co., 1971), pp. 392-394. The variances of the parameter estimates for included variables will be biased upwards, however. Thus, hypothesis tests may be more conservative than indicated.

5. Grossman, *The Demand for Health*, pp. 11-12.

6. Ibid., p. 2. Grossman argues that making P_H a function of H complicates the model but does not alter the basic results.

NOTES TO CHAPTER 3

1. See, for example, C. L. Erhardt and J. E. Berlin, eds., *Mortality and Morbidity in the United States* (Cambridge: Harvard University Press, 1974); Kitagawa and Hauser, *Differential Mortality*, pp. 114-150; and E.S. Colby, "Health Status and the Availability of Health Services System Resources," (D.Sc. dissertation, Johns Hopkins University, 1974).

2. Kitagawa and Hauser, *Differential Mortality*, pp. 114-150, 159-166; Marion E. Altenderfer, "Relationship Between Per Capita Income and Mortality in Cities of 100,000 or More Population," *Public Health Reports* 61 (November 28, 1947). p. 1681; Philip E. Enterline et al., "Death Rates for Coronary Heart Disease in Metropolitan and Other Areas," *Public Health Reports* 75 (August 1960), pp. 759-766; Herbert I. Sauer, "Epidemiology of Cardiovascular Mortality—Geographic and Ethnic," *American Journal of Public Health* 52 (January 1962), pp. 94-105; and Herbert I. Sauer and H. D. Donnell, "Age and Geographic Differences in Death Rates," *Journal of Gerontology* 25 (April 1970), pp. 83-86.

3. Aaron Antonovsky, "Social Class, Life Expectancy, and Overall Mortality," *Milbank Memorial Fund Quarterly* 48 (April 1967), p. 31.

4. Altenderfer, "Relationship Between Per Capita Income and Mortality," p. 1681; T.D. Woolsey, "An Investigation of Low Mortality in Certain Areas," *Public Health Reports* 64 (July 22, 1949), p. 909.

5. Kitagawa and Hauser, *Differential Mortality*, pp. 143-146.

6. Fuchs, *Who Shall Live?*, p. 34; Antonovsky, "Social Class and Overall Mortality," p. 31.

7. Auster et al., "The Production of Health," pp. 430-431; Morris Silver, "An

Econometric Analysis of Spatial Variations in Mortality Rates by Age and Sex," in *Essays in the Economics of Health*, p. 205.

8. Sauer and Donnell, "Age and Geographic Differences in Death Rates," p. 83.

9. B. Benjamin, *Social and Economic Factors Affecting Mortality* (The Hague: Paris, Mouton & Co., 1965); Enterline et al., "Death Rates in Metropolitan and Other Areas," p. 759; and Kitagawa and Hauser, *Differential Mortality*, pp. 120–123.

10. Kitagawa and Hauser, *Differential Mortality*, pp. 152–153.

11. Michael Grossman, "The Correlation between Health and Schooling," in *Household Production and Consumption*, ed. Nestor E. Terleckyj (New York: National Bureau of Economic Research, 1976); Larry M. Manheim, "Health, Health Practices, and Socioeconomic Status: the Role of Education," (Ph.D. dissertation, University of California, Berkeley, 1977), p. 1; and Fuchs, *Who Shall Live?*, pp. 46–47.

12. Fuchs, *Who Shall Live?*, pp. 50–51; Guy H. Orcutt, Stephen D. Franklin, Robert Mendelsohn, and James D. Smith, "Does Your Probability of Death Depend on Your Environment?" *American Economic Review* 67 (February 1977), p. 264; M. Cecil Sheps, "Marriage and Mortality," *American Journal of Public Health* 51 (April 1961), p. 547.

13. Gary D. Friedman, "Cigarette Smoking and Geographic Variations in Coronary Heart Disease Mortality in The United States," *Journal of Chronic Disease* 20 (October 1967), p. 769.; Milicent W. Higgins, Jacob B. Keller, and Helen L. Metzner, "Smoking, Socioeconomic Status and Chronic Respiratory Disease," *American Review of Respiratory Disease* 116 (1977), p. 403; Oscar Auerbach, Cuyler Hammond, and Lawrence Garfinkel, "Changes in Bronchial Epithelium in Relation to Cigarette Smoking," *New England Journal of Medicine* 300 (February 22, 1979), p. 381.

14. Kitagawa and Hauser, *Differential Mortality*, pp. 98–104; Fuchs, *Who Shall Live?*, pp. 35–36.

15. Sauer, "Epidemiology of Cardiovascular Mortality," p. 94; Kitagawa and Hauser, *Differential Mortality*, pp. 157–158.

16. Tavia Gordon, "Mortality Experience Among the Japanese in the United States, Hawaii, and Japan," *Public Health Reports* 72 (June 1957), p. 543.

17. H. A. Schroeder, "Relationship Between Mortality from Cardiovascular Disease and Treated Water Supplies," *Journal of The American Medical Association* 172 (April 23, 1960), p. 1902.

18. Sauer and Donnell, "Age and Geographic Differences in Death Rates," p. 83.

19. Stanley J. States, "Weather and Death in Birmingham, Alabama," *Environmental Research* 12 (1976), p. 340.

20. Lave and Seskin, *Air Pollution and Human Health*, pp. 29–52.

21. Victor Fuchs, "Some Economic Aspects of Mortality in The United States," in *The Economics of Health and Medical Care*, ed. Mark Perlman (New York: John Wiley & Sons, 1974); "The Contribution of Health Services to the American Economy,"; Auster et al., "The Production of Health," p. 412.

22. σ_0 is identified by imposing the restriction that equation (3.2) exhibits constant returns to scale, i.e., the γ_j sum to 1.

23. They cited an earlier paper by Fuchs in which he assumed the share of medical services received by whites is the same as their share of income. However, the coefficients of the modified and unmodified variables were very *similar*. Similar experimentation by the authors produced the same results. Auster et al., "The Production of Health," p. 423.

24. Silver, "Spatial Variations in Mortality Rates," pp. 161–163.

25. Ibid., p. 163.

26. Ibid., p. 195; Auster et al., "The Production of Health," p. 423; Friedman, "Cigarette Smoking and Geographic Variations in Coronary Heart Disease Mortality."

27. Margaret G. Reid, "An Exploration of Conflicting Evidence of Death Rates and Income" (unpublished paper, Department of Economics, University of Chicago, 1976).

28. Ibid., pp. 35–36.

29. Ibid., table 5.

30. Ibid., pp. 32, 41.

31. Orcutt et al., "Does Your Probability of Death Depend on Your Environment?"
p. 260.
32. Ibid., p. 263.
33. Kessner et al., *Infant Death*, p. 177.
34. Ibid.
35. Ibid., pp. 96-122; Sam Shapiro, Edward R. Schlesinger, and Robert E. L. Nesbitt,
Infant, Perinatal, Maternal, and Childhood Mortality in The United States (Cambridge:
Harvard University Press, 1968); and Llad Phillips and Ronald L. Williams, "Perinatal Mortality and Health Services Productivity" (unpublished paper, Community and Organization
Research Institute, University of California, Santa Barbara, 1973), pp. 45-94.
36. Kessner et al., p. 142, 192.
37. Ibid.
38. U.S. Department of Health, Education and Welfare, National Center for Health
Statistics, *A Study of Infant Mortality from Linked Records* (Rockville, Md.: National
Center for Health Statistics, 1972), p. 42.
39. Phillips and Williams, "Perinatal Mortality," pp. 84-86.
40. Ibid.
41. U.S. Department of Health, Education and Welfare, National Center for Health
Statistics, *A Study of Infant Mortality*, p. 58.
42. Shapiro et al., *Infant, Perinatal, Maternal and Childhood Mortality*, pp. 64-65; Edwin W. Jackson and Frank D. Norris, "Impact of Medi-Cal on Perinatal Mortality in
California" (unpublished paper, Department of Public Health, State of California, 1973),
p. 9.
43. Farida K. Shah and Helen Abbey, "Effects of Some Factors on Neonatal and Postneonatal Mortality," *Milbank Memorial Fund Quarterly* 49 (January 1971), p. 43; Carl L.
Erhardt et al., "An Epidemiological Approach to Infant Mortality," *Archives of Environmental Health* 20 (June 1970), pp. 750-751.
44. William I. Barton, "Infant Mortality and Health Insurance Coverage for Maternity
Care," *Inquiry* 9 (Fall 1972): 26; Michael Grossman and Stephen Jacobowitz, "Determinants of Variations in Infant Mortality Rates Among Counties of the United States: The
Roles of Social Programs and Policies" (unpublished paper, National Bureau of Economic
Research, 1981), p. 17 (for whites only).
45. Barton, "Infant Mortality and Health Insurance," pp. 22-25; Kessner et al., *Infant
Death*, pp. 42-45; Grossman and Jacobowitz, "Determinants of Variations in Infant Mortality Rates," p. 17.
46. Jackson and Norris, "The Impact of Medi-Cal on Perinatal Mortality," pp. 11-13;
Erhardt et al., "An Epidemiological Approach to Infant Mortality," p. 753; Beth Berkov
and June Sklar, "Does Illegitimacy Make a Difference? A Study of the Life Chance of Illegitimate Children in California," *Population and Development Review* 2 (June 1976): 215.
47. Shah and Abbey, "Effects of Some Factors on Neonatal and Postneonatal
Mortality," p. 52.
48. Ibid.; Kessner et al., *Infant Death*, p. 1; Erhardt et al., "An Epidemiological Approach to Infant Mortality," p. 747.
49. Jackson and Norris, "Impact of Medi-Cal on Perinatal Mortality," p. 8; Erhardt et
al., "An Epidemiological Approach to Infant Mortality," p. 751.
50. Jackson and Norris, "Impact of Medi-Cal on Perinatal Mortality," p. 26.
51. Kessner et al., *Infant Death*, pp. 1-2.
52. Ronald L. Williams, "Measuring the Effectiveness of Perinatal Medical Care,"
Medical Care 17 (February 1979), p. 98; Williams, "Explaining a Health Care Paradox,"
p. 91.
53. Williams, "Measuring the Effectiveness of Perinatal Medical Care," p. 95.
54. Ibid.
55. Grossman and Jacobowitz, "Determinants of Variations in Infant Mortality Rates,"
pp. 23-28.

NOTES TO CHAPTER 4

1.   Robert M. Kaplan, James W. Bush, and Charles C. Berry, "Health Status: Types of Validity and the Index of Well-Being, *Health Services Research* 11 (Winter 1976), p. 480.

2.   LuAnn Aday, "Criteria for Determining Health Manpower Shortage Areas," in *Workshop on Health Manpower Shortage Areas* (proceedings of a conference sponsored by the U.S. Department of Health, Education and Welfare, Health Resources Administration, Orlando, Florida, December 1976), pp. 111–112; Joel C. Kleinman, Jacob J. Feldman, and Robert H. Mugge, "Geographic Variations in Infant Mortality," *Public Health Reports* 91 (October 1976), p. 423.

3.   For an exception, see Joseph Lipscomb, Lawrence E. Berg, Virginia L. London, and Paul A. Nutting, "Health Status Maximization and Manpower Allocation" (unpublished paper, Center for the Study of Health Policy, Duke University, 1976).

4.   G. A. Whitmore, "The Mortality Component of Health Status Indexes," *Health Services Research* 11 (Winter 1976), p. 373.

5.   R. Kohn, *The Health of the Canadian People* (Ottowa: The Queen's Printer, 1967), pp. 124–125.

6.   Colby, "Health Status and the Availability of Health Services," pp. 226–243.

7.   U.S. Department of Health, Education and Welfare, National Center for Health Statistics, *A Methodological Study of Quality Control Procedures for Mortality Medical Coding*, pp. 2, 4.

8.   See Jack Hadley, "Does Medical Care Affect Health?" final report of Grant No. 5-R01-HS-02790 from the National Center for Health Services Research, USDHHS (Springfield, Va.: National Technical Information Service, 1982), pp. 262–266 for a complete description of how these weights were computed.

9.   See, for example, Sharon R. Henderson, ed., *Profile of Medical Practice 1977* (Chicago: American Medical Association, 1977), p. 147; U.S. Department of Health, Education and Welfare, National Center for Health Statistics, *Utilization of Short-Stay Hospitals, Annual Summary for The United States, 1978* (Hyattsville, Md.: National Center for Health Statistics, 1980), p. 33.

10.   Ralph E. Berry, "On Grouping Hospitals for Economic Analysis," *Inquiry* 10 (December 1973): 9.

11.   Barbara S. Cooper, Nancy L. Worthington, and Paula A. Piro, *Personal Health Care Expenditures by State* (Washington, D.C.: Social Security Administration, 1975), p. 1; U.S. Department of Health, Education and Welfare, Social Security Administration, *Medicare: Health Insurance for the Aged; Amounts Reimbursed by State and County, 1969* (Washington, D.C.: Social Security Administration, 1971), p. 9.

12.   The other components of total medical care spending are long-term care, eyeglasses and appliances, dentists' services, other professional services, and other health services. These are unlikely to be strongly related to variations in mortality rates.

13. $F = 0.19$ with 47 and 1 degrees of freedom.

14.   The t-statistic for β is 51.5 and the R^2 for the equation is 0.98.

15.   Barbara S. Cooper, Nancy L. Worthington, and Mary F. McGee, *Compendium of National Health Expenditures Data* (Washington, D.C.: Social Security Administration, 1973), p. 81.

16.   The medical care component of the CPI varied by about 14 percent for the 22 cities identified separately by the Bureau of Labor Statistics in 1970. The ratios of physicians-to-population and beds-to-population varied by 160 percent and 114 percent, respectively. If, however, prices are positively correlated with expenditures, then the estimates of the Medicare expenditure variable's coefficient will be biased toward zero, thus understating medical care's impact. (I am grateful to Michael Grossman for demonstrating this proposition.) However, a simple regression between the medical care component of the CPI and Medicare expenditures per enrollee for the 22 SMSAs revealed essentially no relationship

between the two (ln CPI = 4.94 − .02·ln MDCREXP, t-statistic = 0.52 for the coefficient of ln MDCREXP). This suggests that there is little bias due to the failure to correct for cross-sectional price differences, although there is no way to know for sure without price data for county groups.

17. Auster et al., pp. 422–424.

NOTES TO CHAPTER 5

1. U.S. Department of Health, Education and Welfare, National Center for Health Statistics, *Vital Statistics of the United States*, 1960 and 1970.

2. Ibid.

3. Omitting initial health state would bias medical care coefficients because of the relationship between health and medical care use.

4. Silver employed a similar approach to control for the effects of psychological tensions by computing the ratio of age-standardized deaths from ulcers to age-standardized deaths from influenza and pneumonia. The denominator was intended to control for variations in the quantity and quality of medical care. Silver, "Spatial Variations in Mortality Rates," pp. 170–171.

5. CIGS is actually defined for the state. However, county groups which cross state borders have CIGS defined as a weighted average of the data for each state, with county populations as weights.

6. Percentages computed from data in the U.S. Department of Health, Education and Welfare, National Center for Health Statistics, *Vital Statistics of the United States 1971*, Vol. II, Part A (Rockville, Md.: 1975), table 1–26.

7. The large coefficient for black males may be due to the concentration of blacks with relatively high mortality rates in the southeastern states, which generally have the highest cigarette sales per capita. This is presumably related to local production and relatively low prices in these states.

8. See Hadley, "Does Medical Care Affect Health?" pp. 267–277 for all coefficients of the cause-specific mortality regressions.

9. Ibid.

10. In 1970, 23.1 percent of males aged 45 to 64, and 37.3 percent of males 65 and older reported never having smoked. The corresponding percentages of females were 54.8 and 81.4, more than twice as great. See U.S. Department of Health, Education and Welfare, National Center for Health Statistics, "Changes in Cigarette Smoking and Current Smoking Practices Among Adults: United States, 1978," *advance data* (September 19, 1979): 2.

11. Lave and Seskin, *Air Pollution and Human Health*, pp. 218–311.

12. Lave and Seskin based their analyses on data for SMSAs. Their model consisted of two basic air pollution variables, sulphate and particulate levels, and four "socioeconomic" variables, population density, percentage 65 and older, percentage nonwhite, and percentage poor. See Lave and Seskin, *Air Pollution and Human Health*, p. 30.

13. Reid, "An Exploration of Conflicting Evidence on Death Rates and Income," p. 36.

NOTES TO CHAPTER 6

1. Phillips and Williams, "Perinatal Mortality and Health Services;" Williams, "Explaining a Health Care Paradox;" Williams, "Measuring the Effectiveness of Perinatal Medical Care."

2. Grossman and Jacobowitz, "Determinants of Variations in Infant Mortality Rates."

3. These data are available on the Area Resource File.

4. Phillips and Williams, "Perinatal Mortality and Health Services;" Shah and Abbey, "Effects of Some Factors on Neonatal and Postneonatal Mortality," p. 54; Kessner et al., *Infant Death*, p. 16.

5. Phillips and Williams, "Perinatal Mortality and Health Services," p. 107; Williams, "Measuring the Effectiveness of Perinatal Medical Care," p. 98.

6. U.S. Department of Health, Education and Welfare, National Center for Health Statistics, *A Study of Infant Mortality from Linked Records*, pp. 31-32.

7. Ibid., p. 15; Kessner et al., *Infant Death*, pp. 97-98.

8. Kessner et al., *Infant Death*, pp. 1, 58; Jackson and Norris, "Impact of Medi-Cal on Perinatal Mortality," p. 8; Erhardt et al., "An Epidemiological Approach to Infant Mortality," p. 751.

9. Phillips and Williams, "Perinatal Mortality and Health Services," p. 128.

10. Grossman and Jacobowitz, "Determinants of Variations in Infant Mortality Rates," p. 17.

11. I am grateful to Michael Grossman and Steven Jacobowitz for providing the information needed to construct these variables.

12. In 1979, these states were Alaska, Arizona, Arkansas, Connecticut, Florida, Georgia, Idaho, Illinois, Indiana, Iowa, Maine, Michigan, Mississippi, Missouri, New Hampshire, New Jersey, North Carolina, Oklahoma, Texas, and Wyoming. (Arizona has no Medicaid program.) Eligibility standards for 1970 are difficult to obtain, but according to the Health Care Financing Administration, provisions regarding coverage of pregnancies have changed very little. See Grossman and Jacobowitz, "Determinants of Variations in Infant Mortality," p. F-3.

13. See U.S. Department of Health, Education and Welfare, Center for Disease Control, *Abortion Surveillance:1970* and subsequent years.

14. The CDC reports data on the number of abortions by women's state of residence. (About 10 percent of reported legal abortions are to women with no known residence.) Some states report data for only a portion of a year. This information was extrapolated to form annual estimates. The total number of abortions over three years, 1971, 1972, and 1973, was summed and divided by the total number of live births. Data on abortions by race and state of residence together are not available.

15. These elasticities imply that a 10 percent increase in physicians increases expenditures by about 5 percent. This proposition will be tested empirically in chapter 8.

16. Kmenta, *Elements of Econometrics*, pp. 389-391.

17. Grossman and Jacobowitz, "Determinants of Variations in Infant Mortality Rates," p. 28.

18. Coefficient estimates are from specification 4 in table 21. Values for males and females were averaged to produce a single value for each race. Elasticities, the percentage change in the dependent variable, infant mortality, for a small percentage change in the independent variable, were then calculated. Since the reliability of the predicted changes decreases the more one moves away from a small range around the observed mean values of the variables, these estimates of relative importance must be treated as crude approximations.

19. See U.S. Department of Health, Education and Welfare, National Center for Health Statistics, *Factors Associated with Low Birth Weight, United States, 1976* (Hyattsville, Md.: National Center for Health Statistics, 1980), for some recent descriptive information.

NOTES TO CHAPTER 7

1. See chapter 3 for a more detailed discussion of the prior research on the relationship between income and mortality.

2. The alternative regression results are available from the author. They are not reported

here because this specification generally performs much less well than the model which includes only the risk and medical care variables. The apparent reason for this is a high degree
of multicollinearity when all variables are included.

3. Auster et al., "The Production of Health;" Silver, "Spatial Variations in Mortality
Rates;" Grossman, "The Correlation Between Health and Schooling."

4. Sheps, "Marriage and Mortality;" Fuchs, *Who Shall Live?*, pp. 50–51.

5. Silver, "Spatial Variations in Mortality Rates," p. 174.

6. Johnston, *Econometric Methods*, p. 169.

7. A priori, if education is hypothesized to be positively related to income but negatively
related to mortality, then omitting education from the regression equation should negatively
bias the income coefficients.

8. Silver, "Spatial Variations in Mortality Rates," pp. 192–193.

NOTES TO CHAPTER 8

1. Hadley, "Alternative Methods of Evaluating Health Manpower Distribution," p.
1056; Aday, "Criteria for Determining Health Manpower Shortage Areas," pp. 111–112.

2. Allowances are made for the numbers of physicians in contiguous counties. See U.S.
Department of Health, Education and Welfare, "Health Manpower Shortage Areas," p.
1588.

3. Fuchs, "Economics, Health, and Post-Industrial Society," p. 155; Glazer, "Paradoxes of Health;" McKinlay and McKinlay, "The Questionable Contribution of Medical
Measures," p 425; Fuchs, *Who Shall Live?*, p. 54; Illich, *Medical Nemesis*, pp. 15–26; Newhouse and Friedlander, "The Relationship Between Medical Resources and Measures of
Health," p. 216.

4. See, for example, G. E. Allen Dever, "An Epidemiological Model for Health Policy
Analysis," *Social Indicators Research* 2 (March 1976):453.

5. If the general form of the health production function is represented by $Y = AX^\beta e^{\gamma Z}$,
then the elasticity of Y with respect to X is β and with respect to Z is γZ, where β and γ are
the estimated parameters of X and Z.

6. This is a necessary assumption since equation (8.3) literally implies that the number
of deaths averted can be made infinitely large by making medical care spending infinitely
large.

7. For simplicity, assume a linear relationship between medical care expenditures and
the supply of physicians. Then the number of needed physicians, ΔMD^*, is equal to $\Delta MC^*/\delta$,
where δ is estimated from the equation $MC_i = \alpha + \delta MD_i$ over i counties.

8. Joel Kleinman, "A New Look at Mortality Indexes with Emphasis on Small Area Estimation," (paper presented at the meeting of the American Statistical Association, Boston,
Mass., August 23, 1976), p. 66.

9. Ronald Andersen, Joanna Kravits, Odin W. Andersen, and Joan Daley, *Expenditures
for Personal Health Services: National Trends and Variations 1953–1970* (Rockville, Md.:
Bureau of Health Services Research and Development, 1973) pp. 1–2.

10. Cooper et al., *Compendium of National Health Expenditures*, p. 81.

11. Andersen et al., *Expenditures for Personal Health Services*, p. 65.

12. Ibid., p. 36.

13. This mortality rate is about three times larger than that for the entire population. This
is because deaths among the 12 cohorts in the study account for approximately 90 percent of all
deaths, while the cohorts' population comprise only 35 percent of all people.

14. Results for rank-order correlations were very similar.

15. For the 500 counties with the largest values of DAMC the correlations between DAMC
and POPPC and POPMD are −0.01 and 0.05, respectively. For the 500 counties with the
largest values of POPMD, the correlations are 0.20 and 0.24, about the same as for all counties.

16. This is a standard adjustment for heteroskedasticity, which is very common when the
observational units differ so dramatically in size.

17.   U.S. Department of Commerce, Bureau of the Census, *Current Population Reports,* Series P-60, No. 80, "Income in 1970 of Families and Persons in The United States," Washington, D.C.: U.S. Government Printing Office, 1971, pp. 17, 31.

18.   Kenneth E. Warner, "The Effects of the Anti-Smoking Campaign on Cigarette Consumption," *American Journal of Public Health* 67 (July 1977):645; James L. Hamilton, "The Demand for Cigarettes: Advertising, The Health Scare, and The Cigarette Advertising Ban," *The Review of Economics and Statistics* 54 (November 1972):401.

19.   Hamilton, "The Demand for Cigarettes," p. 407, table 4, line 8.

20.   Warner, "The Effects of the Anti-Smoking Campaign," p. 648.

21.   Kmenta, *Elements of Econometrics,* p. 393.

22.   Hamilton, "The Demand for Cigarettes," p. 408.

23.   U.S. Department of Health, Education and Welfare, National Center for Health Statistics, "Cigarette Smoking in The United States, 1970," *Monthly Vital Statistics Report* 21, Supplement (June 2, 1972), p. 4.

24.   U.S. Department of Health, Education and Welfare, National Center for Health Statistics, "Changes in Cigarette Smoking and Current Smoking Practices Among Adults: United States, 1978," *advancedata* 52 (September 19, 1979), p. 6.

25.   U.S. Department of Commerce, Bureau of the Census, Series P-60, No. 80, "Income in 1970 of Families." Aggregate family income is from p. 17; income of unrelated individuals is estimated from p. 28.

NOTES TO APPENDIX A

1.   U.S. Department of Commerce, Bureau of the Census, *Public Use Samples of Basic Records from the 1970 Census: Description and Technical Documentation* (Washington, D.C.: Bureau of the Census, 1972), pp. 4–5.

2.   Auster et al., "The Production of Health," p. 430.

3.   More formally, if the mortality rate is thought of as the probability of dying, then its variance is given by $M(1 - M)/N$, where M is the probability of dying and N is the size of the population. Clearly, the larger N is the smaller variance.

4.   Johnston, *Econometric Methods* (New York: McGraw-Hill Book Co., 1972), second edition, p. 219.

5.   Auster et al., "The Production of Health.;" Silver, "Spatial Variations in Mortality Rates;" Williams, "Explaining a Health Care Paradox;" Grossman and Jacobowitz, "Determinants of Variations in Infant Mortality Rates."

6.   Kmenta, *Elements of Econometrics,* pp. 302–303.

7.   Lave and Seskin made a similar assumption in their study of the impact of air pollution on mortality rates. See Lave and Seskin, *Air Pollution and Human Health,* p. 22.

8.   Silver, "Spatial Variations in Mortality Rates," pp. 170–171.

9.   See Hadley, "Does Medical Care Affect Health?" pp. 262–266 for details on the construction of cohort-specific estimates.

10.   Johnston, *Econometric Methods,* p. 219.

BIBLIOGRAPHY

Aday, LuAnn. "Criteria for Determining Health Manpower Shortage Areas." In *Proceedings of the Workshop on Health Manpower Shortage Areas, November 8-10, 1976 Orlando, Florida.* Washington, D.C.: Moshman Associates, Inc., December 1976.

Altenderfer, Marion E. "Relationship Between Per Capita Income and Mortality, in the Cities of 100,000 or more Population." *Public Health Reports* 62 (November 28, 1947): 1681-1691.

Andersen, Ronald; Kravits, Joanna; and Anderson, Odin W. *Expenditures for Personal Health Services: National Trends and Variations, 1953-1970.* Rockville, Md.: Bureau of Health Services Research and Evaluation, 1973.

_____eds. *Equity in Health Services: Empirical Analyses in Social Policy.* Cambridge: Ballinger Publishing Co., 1975.

Antonovsky, Aaron. "Social Class, Life Expectancy and Overall Mortality." *Milbank Memorial Fund Quarterly* 48, part I (April 1967): 31-73.

Auerbach, Oscar; Hammond, E. Cuyler; and Garfinkel, Lawrence. "Changes in Bronchial Epithelium in Relation to Cigarette Smoking, 1955-1960 vs. 1970-77." *The New England Journal of Medicine* 300 (February 22, 1979): 381-386.

Auster, Richard; Leveson, Irving; and Sarachek, Deborah. "The Production of Health, An Exploratory Study." *Journal of Human Resources* 4 (Fall 1969): 411-436.

Barton, William I. "Infant Mortality and Health Insurance Coverage for Maternity Care." *Inquiry* 9 (September 1972): 16-29.

Benjamin, B. *Social and Economic Factors Affecting Mortality.* The Hague: Paris, Mouton & Co., 1965.

Berkov, Beth, and Sklar, June. "Does Illegitimacy Make a Difference? A Study of Life Chances of Illegitimate Children of California." *Population and Development Review* 2 (June 1976): 201-217.

Berry, Ralph E. "On Grouping Hospitals for Economic Analysis." *Inquiry* 10 (December 1973): 5-12.

Bissel, H. Preston; Foust, J. Brady; and Loomba, Bodh. "Spatial Aspects of Mortality in the United States." Council of Planning Librarians: Exchange Bibliography no. 439. Monticello, Ill.: Council of Planning Librarians, 1973. (Unpublished.)

The Blue Sheet. "Summary of HEW Health Planning Goals." 22 (October 31, 1979) pp. S-17,18.

Blum, Henrik L. *Planning for Health.* New York: Human Sciences Press, Behavioral Publications Inc., 1974.

231

Brook, Robert H.; Davies, Allyson Ross; and Kamberg, Caren J. *Selected Reflections on Quality of Medical Care Evaluation in the 1980s.* Santa Monica: Rand Corporation, 1979.

Colby, Edward S. "Health Status and the Availability of Health Services System Resources." Sc. D. dissertation, Johns Hopkins University, 1974.

Cooper, Barbara S.; Worthington, Nancy L.; and McGee, Mary F. *Compendium of National Health Expenditures Data.* Washington, D.C.: Social Security Administration, 1972.

_____; and Piro, Paula A. *Personal Health Care Expenditures by States.* Washington, D.C.: Social Security Administration, 1975.

Dever, G. E. A. "An Epidemiological Model for Health Policy Analysis." *Social Indicators Research* 2 (March 1976): 453-466.

Enterline, Philip E., and Stewart, William, H. "Geographic Patterns in Deaths from Coronary Heart Disease." *Public Health Reports* 71 (September 1956): 849.

_____; Rikli, A. E.; Sauer, H. I.; and Hyman, M. "Death Rates for Coronary Heart Disease in Metropolitan and Other Areas." *Public Health Reports* 75 (August 1960): 759-766.

Erhardt, Carl L.; Abramson, Harold; Pakter, Jean; and Nelson, Frieda. "An Epidemiological Approach to Infant Mortality." *Archives of Environmental Health* 20 (June 1970): 743-757.

_____, and Berlin, J. E., eds. *Mortality and Morbidity in the United States.* Cambridge: Harvard University Press, 1974.

Fishman, Alfred P. "How Safe Can Cigarettes Be?" *The New England Journal of Medicine* 300 (February 22, 1979): 428-430.

Friedman, Gary D. "Cigarette Smoking and Geographic Variations in Coronary Heart Disease Mortality in The United States." *Journal of Chronic Disease* 20 (October 1967): 769-779.

Fuchs, Victor R. "Economics, Health and Post-Industrial Society." *Milbank Memorial Fund Quarterly* 57 (Spring 1979): 153-182.

_____*Who Shall Live?* New York: Basic Books Inc., 1974.

_____"Some Economic Aspects of Mortality in the United States." In *The Economics of Health and Medical Care,* pp. 174-93. Edited by Mark Perlman. New York: John Wiley & Sons, 1974.

_____, ed. *Essays in the Economics of Health and Medical Care.* New York: National Bureau of Economic Research, 1972.

_____, and Kramer, Marcia J. *Determinants of Expenditures for Physicians' Services in the United States, 1948-1968.* Rockville, Md.: U.S. Department of Health, Education and Welfare, 1972.

Gibson, Robert M., and Mueller, Marjorie Smith. "National Health Expenditures, Fiscal Year 1976." *Social Security Bulletin* 40, no. 4, (April 1977): 3-22.

Glazer, Nathan. "Paradoxes of Health Care." *The Public Interest* 22 (Winter 1971): 62-77.

Gordon, Tavia. "Mortality Experience Among the Japanese in the United States, Hawaii, and Japan." *Public Health Reports* 72 (June 1957): 543-553.

Grossman, Michael. "The Correlation between Health and Schooling." In *Household Production and Consumption,* pp. 147-211. Edited by Nestor E. Tenleckyj. New York: National Bureau of Economic Research, 1976.

_____*The Demand for Health: A Theoretical and Empirical Investigation.* New York: National Bureau of Economic Research, 1972.

_____,and Benham, Lee. "Health, Hours and Wages." In *The Economics of Health and Medical Care,* pp. 205–33. Edited by Mark A. Perlman. New York: John Wiley & Sons, 1974.

_____, and Jacobowitz, Steven. "Determinants of Variations in Infant Mortality Rates Among Counties of the United States: The Roles of Social Policies and Programs." National Bureau of Economic Research, 1981. (Unpublished.)

Hadley, Jack. "Does Medical Care Affect Health?" "Final report of Grant No. 5-R01-HS-02790 from the National Center for Health Services Research, U.S. Department of Health and Human Services. Springfield, Va.: National Technical Information Service, 1982.

_____. "Alternative Methods of Evaluating Health Manpower Distribution." *Medical Care* 17 (October 1979): 1054–1060.

Hamilton, James L. "The Demand for Cigarettes: Advertising, the Health Scare, and the Cigarette Advertising Ban." *Review of Economics and Statistics* 54 (November 1972): 401–411.

Henderson, Sharon R., ed. *Profile of Medical Practice, 1977.* Chicago: American Medical Association, 1977.

Higgins, Millicent W.; Keller, Jacob B.; and Metzner, Helen L. "Smoking, Socioeconomic Status, and Chronic Respiratory Disease." *American Review of Respiratory Disease* 116 (1977): 403–410.

Illich, Ivan. *Medical Nemesis.* New York: Pantheon Books, Random House, 1976.

Jackson, Edwin W., and Norris, Frank D. "Impact of Medi-Cal on Perinatal Mortality." State of California, Department of Public Health, 1973. (Unpublished.)

Johnston, J. *Econometric Methods.* 2nd ed. New York: McGraw-Hill Book Co., 1972.

Kaplan, Robert M.; Bush, J. W.; and Berry, Charles C. "Health Status: Types of Validity and the Index of Well-being." *Health Services Research* 11 (Winter 1976): 478–507.

Kessner, David M.; Singer, James; Kalk, Carolyn E.; and Schlesinger, Edward R. *Infant Death: An Analysis by Maternal Risk and Health Care,* Vol. 1. Washington, D. C.: National Academy of Sciences, 1973.

Kitagawa, Evelyn M., and Hauser, Philip M. *Differential Mortality in the United States.* Cambridge: Harvard University Press, 1973.

Klarman, Herbert E. *The Economics of Health.* New York: Columbia University Press, 1965.

Kleinman, Joel. "A New Look at Mortality Indexes with Emphasis on Small Area Estimation," Paper presented at the Contributed Paper Session of the American Statistical Association, Boston, Mass., August 23, 1976.

_____; Feldman, Jacob J.; and Mugge, Robert H. "Geographic Variations in Infant Mortality." *Public Health Reports* 91 (September–October 1976): 423–432.

Kmenta, Jan. *Elements of Econometrics.* New York: Macmillan Publishing Co., Inc., 1971.

Kohn, R. *The Health of the Canadian People.* Ottawa: The Queen's Printer, 1967.

Lave, Lester B., and Seskin, Eugene P. *Air Pollution and Human Health.* Baltimore: Johns Hopkins University Press, 1977.

Lerner, Monroe, and Stutz, Richard. "Mortality by Socioeconomic Status, 1959-61 and 1969-71." *Maryland State Medical Journal* 27 (December 1978): 35-42.

Lipscomb, Joseph; Berg, Lawrence E.; London, Virginia L.; and Nutting, Paul A. "Health Status Maximization and Manpower Allocation." Institute of Policy Sciences and Public Affairs Working Paper Series, no. 9761. Durham, N.C.: Duke University, September 1976. (Unpublished.)

Manheim, Larry M. "Health, Health Practices, and Socioeconomic Status: The Role of Education." Ph.D. dissertation, University of California, Berkeley, 1977.

McKinlay, John B., and McKinlay, Sonja M. "The Questionable Contribution of Medical Measures to the Decline of Mortality in the United States in the Twentieth Century." *Milbank Memorial Fund Quarterly* 55 (Summer 1977): 405-429.

Newhouse, Joseph P., and Friedlander, Lindy J. "The Relationship Between Medical Resources and Measures of Health: Some Additional Evidence." *Journal of Human Resources* 15 (Spring 1980): 200-218.

Orcutt, Guy H.; Franklin, Stephen D.; Mendelsohn, Robert; and Smith, James D. "Does Your Probability of Death Depend on Your Environment?" *American Economic Review* 67 (February 1977): 260-264.

Phillips, Llad, and Williams, Ronald L. "Final Report: Perinatal Mortality and Health Services Productivity." University of California, Santa Barbara. Community and Organization Research Institute. Santa Barbara, 1973. (Unpublished.)

Reid, Margaret G. "An Exploration of Conflicting Evidence of Death Rates and Income." University of Chicago. Chicago, 1976. (Unpublished.)

Rutstein, David D.; Berenberg, William; Chalmers, Thomas C.; Child, Charles G.; Fishman, Alfred P.; and Perrin, Edward B. "Measuring the Quality of Medical Care." (Tables Revised, September 1, 1977). *New England Journal of Medicine* 294 (March 11, 1976): 582-588.

Sauer, Herbert I. "Epidemiology of Cardiovascular Mortality—Geographic and Ethnic." *American Journal of Public Health* 52 (January 1962): 94-105.

————, and Donnell, H. D. "Age and Geographic Differences in Death Rates." *Journal of Gerontology* 25 (April 1970): 83-86.

Schroeder, Henry A. "Relation Between Mortality from Cardiovascular Disease and Treated Water Supplies." *Journal of the American Medical Association* 172 (April 23, 1960): 1902-1908.

Shah, Farida, and Abbey, Helen. "Effects of Some Factors on Neonatal and Postneonatal Mortality." *Milbank Memorial Fund Quarterly* 49 (January 1971): 33-57.

Shapiro, Sam; Schlesinger, Edward R.; and Nesbitt, Robert E. L., Jr. *Infant, Perinatal, Maternal, and Childhood Mortality in the United States.* Cambridge: Harvard University Press, 1968.

Sheps, Mindel C. "Marriage and Mortality." *American Journal of Public Health* 51 (April 1961): 547-555.

Silver, Morris. "An Econometric Analysis of Spatial Variations in Mortality Rates." In *Essays in the Economics of Health*, pp. 161-227. Edited by Victor R. Fuchs. New York: National Bureau of Economic Research, 1972.

States, Stanley J. "Weather and Death in Birmingham, Alabama." *Environmental Research* 12 (1976): 340-354.

Tobacco Tax Council, Inc. *The Tax Burden on Tobacco, Historical Compilation,* Vol. 12. Richmond, Virginia: Tobacco Tax Council, 1977.

U.S., Department of Commerce, Bureau of the Census. "Income in 1970 of Families and Persons in the United States." *Current Population Reports,* Series P-60, No. 80. Washington, D.C.: U.S. Government Printing Office, 1971.

U.S., Department of Health, Education and Welfare, Health Care Financing Administration. "National Health Expenditures and Related Measures." *Health Care Financing Trends* (Fall 1979).

U.S., Department of Health, Education and Welfare, National Center for Health Statistics. *A Methodological Study of Quality Control Procedures for Mortality Medical Coding.* DHEW Publication No. (PHS) 80-1355. Hyattsville, Md.: National Center for Health Statistics, March 1980.

———. *Factors Associated with Low Birth Weight, United States, 1976.* Hyattsville, Md.: National Center for Health Statistics, April 1980.

———. "Changes in Cigarette Smoking Practices Among Adults: United States, 1978." *advance data* 52 (September 19, 1979).

———. *Utilization of Short-Stay Hospitals, Annual Summary for the United States, 1978.* Hyattsville, Md.: National Center for Health Statistics, 1978.

———. *State Estimates of Disability and Utilization of Medical Services: United States, 1974-76.* Hyattsville, Md.: National Center for Health Statistics, 1978.

———. *Infant Mortality Rates: Relationship with Mother's Reproductive History.* DHEW Publication No. (HSM) 73-1976. Rockville, Md.: National Center for Health Statistics, April 1973.

———. *A Study of Infant Mortality From Linked Records, by Birthweight, Period of Gestation and Other Variables.* DHEW Publication No. (PHS) 79-1055. Rockville, Md.: National Center for Health Statistics, 1972.

———. *Infant Mortality Rates: Socioeconomic Factors.* DHEW Publication No. (HSM) 72-1045. Rockville, Md.: National Center for Health Statistics, March 1972.

———. "Cigarette Smoking in the United States, 1970." *Monthly Vital Statistics Report* 21 (Supplement, June 2, 1972).

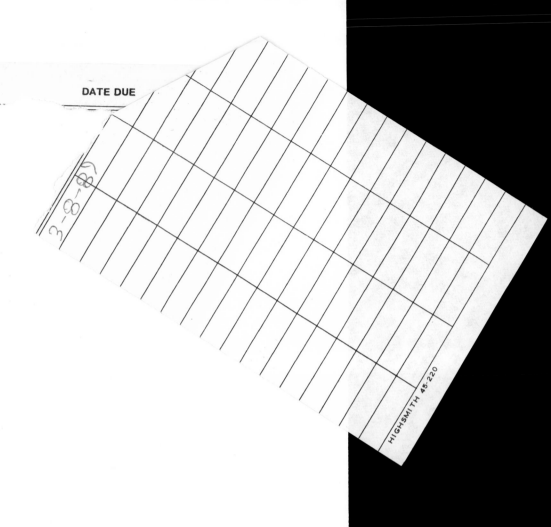